Monitoring Mechanical Ventilation Using Ventilator Waveforms

Jean-Michel Arnal

Monitoring Mechanical Ventilation Using Ventilator Waveforms

With Contribution by Robert Chatburn

Springer

Jean-Michel Arnal
Service de Réanimation
Polyvalente
Hopital Sainte Musse
Toulon, France

Applied Research and New
Technology
Hamilton Medical AG
Bonaduz, Switzerland

With contribution by Robert Chatburn

ISBN 978-3-319-58654-0 ISBN 978-3-319-58655-7 (eBook)
https://doi.org/10.1007/978-3-319-58655-7

Library of Congress Control Number: 2017957539

Printed on acid-free paper

This Springer imprint is published by Springer Nature
The registered company is Springer International Publishing AG
The registered company address is: Gewerbestrasse 11, 6330 Cham, Switzerland

Foreword

The study of mechanical ventilation, medicine in general, and perhaps our whole society is struggling under an ominous threat: explosive complexity in technology. It is a threat for the simple reason that the resources spent on technological complexity have increased exponentially over time, while simultaneously, the resources spent on tools to understand and effectively use this technology is holding a constant rate (at best). If you can visualize the graph I have suggested, it would indicate a growing knowledge gap on the part of clinicians and, in particular, physicians using mechanical ventilators. I have been teaching mechanical ventilation for nearly four decades, and I have yet to meet a physician who was provided any substantial training about mechanical ventilation in medical school. This seems astounding, given that life support technologies (resuscitation, intubation, and mechanical ventilation) are critical skills needed by most patients who must endure a stay in an intensive care unit.

As with any advanced medical skill, the road to mastery of mechanical ventilation can be viewed as a hierarchy of specific accomplishments. First, one needs to understand the terminology and then how this terminology is used to describe the technology in terms of both theoretical concepts and a formal taxonomy. In this case, the taxonomy helps us identify modes of ventilation, independent of the names manufacturers coin to sell products. Next, we need to appreciate the specific technological capabilities that different ventilators offer and be able to sort them into advantages and disadvantages. Finally, we need to be able to assess the goal of ventilation for a particular patient (safety, comfort, or liberation) and then match the available technology to the patient's needs. This, of course, involves selecting the most appropriate mode of ventilation. But perhaps the more challenging problem is to select the optimum settings. This is an ongoing challenge because of the constantly changing nature of a patient's condition. Optimizing settings requires that the clinician understand the intricacies of patient-ventilator interactions, particularly in terms of the measured variables as they are displayed by ventilator graphics. In my experience, this is the most difficult skill for clinicians to master. Not only does it require a certain level of theoretical knowledge, but it also requires experience at the bedside.

That brings us to the purpose of this handbook. Consistent, accurate, and practical information regarding ventilator waveform analysis is surprisingly difficult to obtain in book form. To address the need, the author of this book has combined his decades of experience in clinical practice, engineering, and medical education to provide a quick reference work for clinicians at the bedside. The information is presented in short summaries organized in a way that facilitates understanding, using actual ventilator displays and real problems encountered in the daily practice of mechanical ventilation. Each section has a set of self-study questions.

Understanding of the concepts in this resource is a key step in the mastery of the art and science of mechanical ventilation. But remember, knowledge is no substitute for wisdom.

Health and Peace

May, 2017

R. L. Chatburn, MHHS, RRT-NPS, FAARC
Respiratory Institute, Cleveland Clinic
Cleveland, OH, USA

Lerner College of Medicine of Case
Western Reserve University
Cleveland, OH, USA

Preface

Waveforms are widely available on mechanical ventilator screens and provide clinicians with both precise and important information at the bedside. Ventilator waveforms are produced from measurements of airway pressure and flow, and combine curves and loops. The pressure and flow curves should be interpreted together using different time scales. They represent the interaction between the ventilator and the patient's respiratory mechanics described by the equation of motion. This book is intended for bedside clinicians wanting to assess the effect of ventilator settings on their patients, in order to protect the lung and optimize patient-ventilator synchrony.

The first chapter introduces the basics of respiratory mechanics and interpreting curves. The two main characteristics of respiratory mechanics are compliance and resistance, both of which can be calculated directly from the ventilator waveforms using occlusion maneuvers. The product of compliance and resistance is the time constant, which represents the dynamic respiratory mechanics and is thus very useful at the bedside. Chapters 2–4 detail curves in control modes, during expiration, and in spontaneous modes. In control modes, pressure and flow curves are used to assess respiratory mechanics and measure plateau pressure as a substitute of alveolar pressure. Monitoring of expiration is reliant mainly on the flow curve, which in turn depends on the expiratory time constant. Therefore, monitoring of the expiratory flow provides us with information about the patient's respiratory mechanics and enables detection of dynamic hyperinflation. In pressure support modes, the flow curve informs us about the patient effort and patient-ventilator synchrony, while observation of both the flow and pressure curves helps us to optimize the inspiratory trigger setting, the rise time, and the expiratory trigger setting. Chapter 5 looks at curves in noninvasive ventilation and two particularities of NIV, unintentional leaks and upper airway obstruction, which can also be detected on the flow curve. Chapter 6 covers quasi-static pressure-volume loops used mainly in severe hypoxemic patients to assess lung recruitability, while Chap. 7 describes an esophageal pressure curve that can be added to the airway pressure and flow for several useful applications, such as assessing the risk of stress and atelectrauma. The esophageal pressure can also be used to display a transpulmonary pressure-volume curve and to assess the transpulmonary pressure applied during a recruitment maneuver. In spontaneously breathing patients, the esophageal pressure curve shows the patient effort and patient-ventilator synchrony.

Each page contains a short explanation, a figure, and a quiz question. In most instances, the figures are screenshots taken from real patients with normal artifacts present. The pressure curve is displayed in yellow, and the flow curve in pink. For each question, there is only one correct answer and you will find the answers and comments at the end of each chapter.

I trust you will find the information contained in this book both interesting and useful in your daily work. Should you have comments or additional questions about any of the contents, please don't hesitate to contact me.

Toulon, France Jean-Michel Arnal

Acknowledgments

The author thanks Dr. Aude Garnero and Mrs. Caroline Huber-Brown for their invaluable support in reviewing and editing the manuscript.

Contents

Abbreviations

ARDS	Acute respiratory disease syndrome
C_{DYN}	Dynamic compliance of the respiratory system
CO_2	Carbon dioxide
COPD	Chronic obstructive respiratory disease
C_{RS}	Compliance of the respiratory system; $C_{RS} = V_T/\Delta P$
C_{STAT}	Static compliance of the respiratory system
E_{RS}	Elastance of the respiratory system; $E_{RS} = \Delta P/V_T$
ET	Endotracheal
ETS	Expiratory trigger sensitivity
HME	Heat and moisture exchanger
I:E	Inspiratory-expiratory time ratio
NIV	Noninvasive ventilation
P_1	Initial pressure
P_A	Alveolar pressure
P_{AW}	Airway pressure
PC	Pressure control mode
PEEP	Positive end-expiratory pressure
AutoPEEP	Intrinsic PEEP
$PEEP_{TOT}$	Total PEEP measured by an end-expiratory occlusion; $PEEP_{TOT}$ = PEEP + AutoPEEP
P_{EL}	Elastic pressure; the amount of pressure to overcome elastic forces
P_{ES}	Esophageal pressure
P_{INSP}	Preset inspiratory pressure
P_{MUS}	Pressure generated by the patient's muscles
P_{PEAK}	Peak pressure
P_{PLAT}	Plateau pressure measured by an end-inspiratory occlusion
P_{RES}	Resistive pressure: the amount of pressure to overcome resistance

PS	Pressure support mode
P_{TA}	Transalveolar pressure; $P_{TA} = P_A - P_{ES}$
P_{TP}	Transpulmonary pressure; $P_{TP} = P_{AW} - P_{ES}$
PV	Pressure-volume
R_{ADD}	Additional resistance
RC_{EXP}	Expiratory time constant
RC_{INSP}	Inspiratory time constant
R_{EXP}	Expiratory resistance
R_{INSP}	Inspiratory resistance
R_{MAX}	Maximum resistance
R_{MIN}	Minimum resistance
VAC	Volume assist control mode
VC	Volume control mode
V_T	Tidal volume
ΔP_{TA}	Transpulmonary driving pressure
ΔP	Airway driving pressure
ΔV	Change in volume

List of Videos

Electronic supplementary material is available in the online version of the related chapter on SpringerLink: http://link.springer.com/

Chapter 1
Basics

1.1 What Is a Curve?

Curves (also known as scalars) are real-time graphical representations of a variable (*pressure, flow*, or *volume*) according to time.

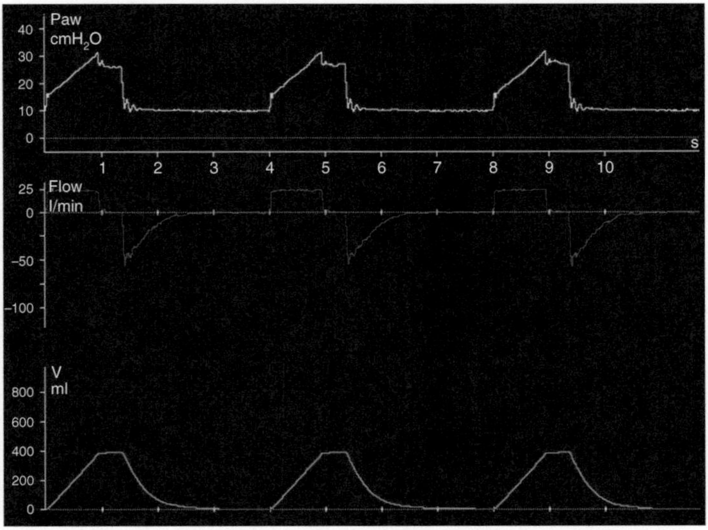

J.-M. Arnal, *Monitoring Mechanical Ventilation Using Ventilator Waveforms*, https://doi.org/10.1007/978-3-319-58655-7_1

On a curve, the x-axis always represents:

1. Flow
2. Pressure
3. Volume
4. Time
5. Points north

1.2 Which Curves Are Relevant?

Ventilators measure airway pressure and airway flow. Volume is derived from the flow measurement. *Pressure and flow* provide all the information necessary to explain the physical interaction between ventilator and patient.

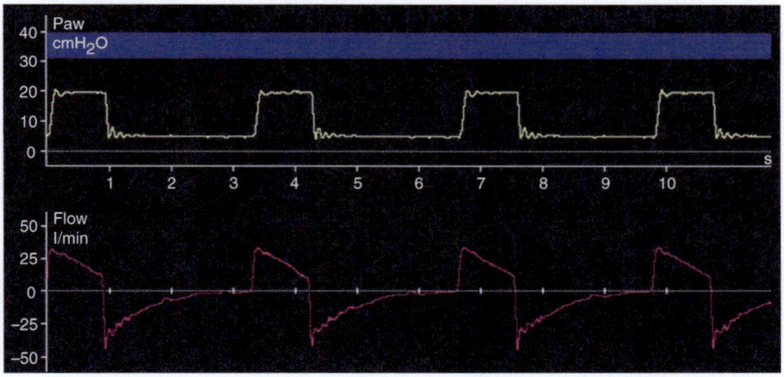

Monitoring of mechanical ventilation relies on the analysis of:

1. The pressure curve
2. The flow curve
3. The volume curve
4. The interactions among pressure and flow
5. The temperature curve

1.3 What Is a Loop?

A loop is a real-time graphical representation of *two variables* (pressure, flow, or volume) plotted against one another. One loop displays the values for one breath.

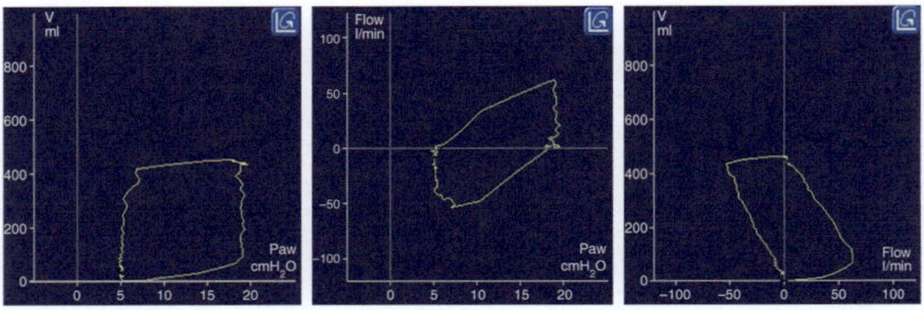

In comparison to curves, loops show:

1. The interaction between variables
2. The same information
3. More information about flow
4. More information about time
5. The dark side of the moon

1.4 Pressure Curve

The pressure curve is always *positive* during mechanical ventilation. Baseline pressure above zero appears when PEEP is applied and assisted inspiration (i.e., work done by the ventilator on the patient) is shown as an increase in pressure above PEEP during volume delivery.

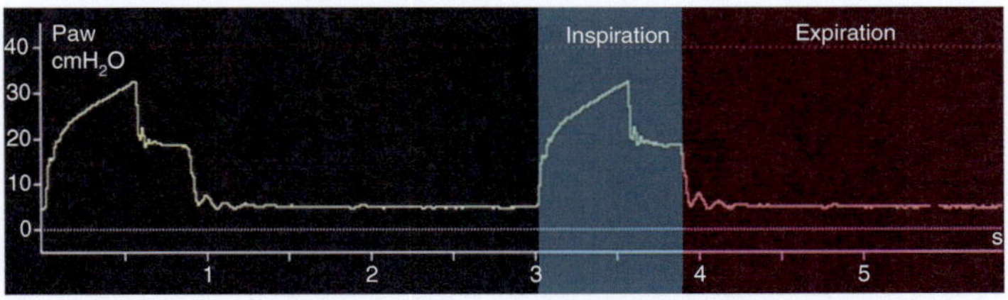

The pressure curve represents the pressure:

1. At the flow outlet of the ventilator
2. At the proximal airway
3. At the end of the endotracheal tube
4. In the alveoli
5. At sea level

1.5 Flow Curve

Flow is displayed above the zero flow line, i.e., *positive values, during inspiration* (when gas travels from the ventilator to the patient), and below the zero flow line, i.e., *negative values, during expiration* (when gas travels from the patient back to the ventilator). If there is a pause at the end of inspiration, it is considered as part of the inspiratory time. The inspiratory time is therefore measured from the beginning of positive flow to the beginning of negative flow.

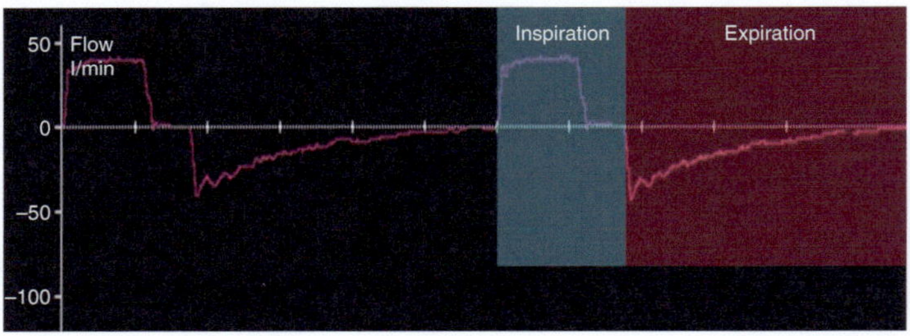

Flow is:

1. Always positive
2. Always negative
3. Positive or negative depending on mode of ventilation
4. Positive or negative depending on the breath phase
5. Dependent on the wind direction

1.6 Volume Curve

Volume is usually not measured directly (except for piston ventilators), but is *derived from the flow* measurement as the area under the flow-time curve. The upslope represents inspiratory volume, while the downslope represents expiratory volume. Any plateau between the two represents an end-inspiratory pause (optional). Inspiratory and expiratory tidal volumes may differ slightly due to the accuracy of the flow measurement, as well as differences in the temperature or humidity of gas. A large discrepancy between inspired and expired tidal volumes may suggest gas leakage. However, the volume display is usually reset to zero at the end of expiration so that errors do not accumulate graphically.

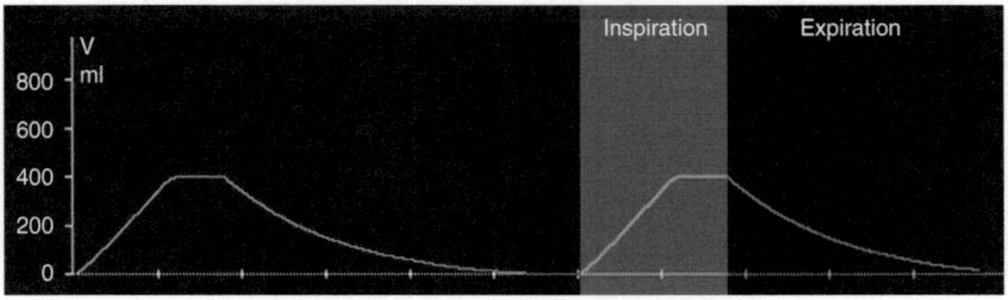

On the volume curve:

1. A volume increase is always linear
2. A volume increase is always exponential
3. The shape of the inspiratory volume waveform is dependent on the shape of the inspiratory flow waveform
4. A volume decrease is exponential if expiration is active
5. Inspiratory and expiratory volume are always the same

1.7 Time Scale

The time scale is often set automatically at 10 s per epoch in order to analyze 3 or 4 breaths. However, it may be useful to manually zoom out to 30 s or more for repetitive events such as obstructive apnea or Cheyne-Stokes respiration or to zoom in for a detailed assessment of patient-ventilator synchrony.

By freezing the curve, it is possible to observe one single event. Using the cursor, pressure or flow can be measured at any point, and synchronization between pressure and flow can be assessed.

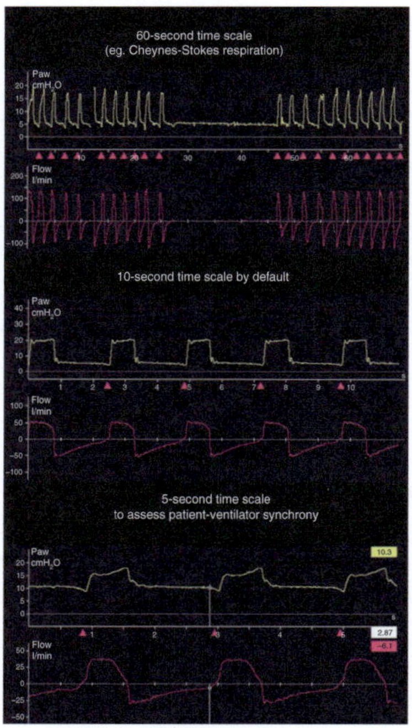

The time scale:

1. Is not really important
2. Is not the same for pressure, volume, and flow
3. Can be manually adjusted depending on requirements
4. Depends on the respiratory rate
5. Depends on ventilation mode

1.8 Mandatory and Triggered Breaths

A *spontaneous breath* is one for which inspiration is both triggered (started) and cycled (stopped) by the patient. A *mandatory breath* is one for which inspiration is either ventilator triggered or ventilator cycled (or both). This is a key concept in understanding the taxonomy for modes of ventilation. A breath triggered by the patient shows a pressure deflection below the baseline (or a flow deflection above baseline) just before the rise in pressure indicating the start of inspiratory flow from the ventilator. Here patient triggering is indicated by the small triangles below each breath. Absence of these triangles indicates ventilator (i.e., time) triggering.

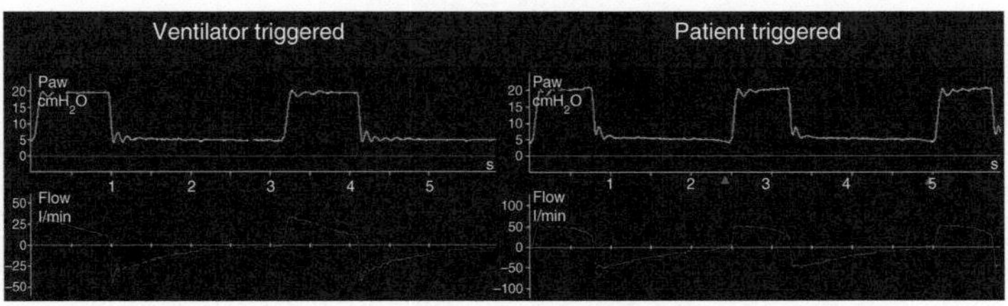

When the patient triggers the breath:

1. There is always a delay between patient effort and flow delivery
2. A small increase in flow before triggering indicates a flow-triggering system
3. A short period of flow at zero before triggering indicates a pressure-triggering system
4. Pressure deflection is deeper if the patient has a high respiratory drive
5. All are correct

1.9 Static Respiratory Mechanics

The respiratory system can be simplified using a linear one-compartment model, which comprises a *tube* representing the airways and a *balloon* representing the alveoli and the chest wall. To ventilate such a system, there are two main forces that oppose inflation of the balloon:

1. The impedance to flow, which represents resistance of the airways:
   - Resistance = Δ pressure/flow
2. The impedance to volumetric expansion, which represents compliance of the lung and chest wall:
   - Compliance = Δ volume/Δ pressure
   - Elastance = Δ pressure/Δ volume

Note that the linear one-compartment model does not take into account the fact that resistance and compliance are not constant in the case of lung and chest-wall disease; instead they exhibit a flow and volume dependency. It also does not include the effects of inertia, which are small for normal respiratory frequencies. Most ventilators ignore these details in their calculations for resistance and compliance.

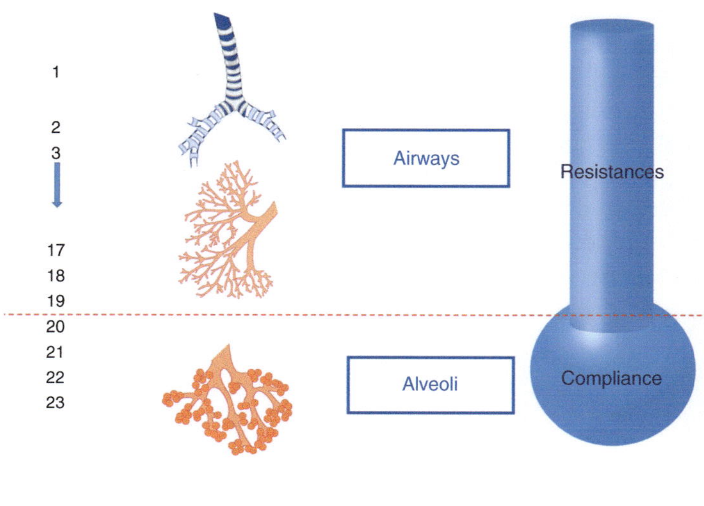

The two main characteristics of respiratory mechanics during mechanical ventilation are:

1. Lung heterogeneity
2. Airway resistance
3. Inertia
4. Compliance of the lung and chest wall
5. Both 2 and 4

1.10 Equation of Motion in Passive Patients

The graphical, single-compartment model shown above has a *mathematical correlate*, called the equation of motion for the respiratory system. It is essentially a force balance equation. At any point in time during inspiration, airway pressure (P_{AW}) is the sum of:

- The starting pressure: Total PEEP ($PEEP_{TOT}$)
- The resistive pressure (P_{RES}): Pressure to overcome the inspiratory resistance. P_{RES} is the product of inspiratory resistance and inspiratory flow.
- The elastic pressure (P_{EL}): Pressure to overcome the lung and chest-wall compliance. P_{EL} is the ratio of tidal volume to respiratory-system compliance:

$$P_{AW} = PEEP_{TOT} + P_{RES} + P_{EL}$$

$$= PEEP_{TOT} + (\text{tidal volume} / \text{compliance}) + (\text{flow} \times \text{resistance})$$

or

$$P_{AW} - PEEP_{TOT} = (\text{tidal volume} / \text{compliance}) + (\text{flow} \times \text{resistance})$$

where $PEEP_{TOT}$ is the pressure in the lungs at the end of the expiratory time, which depends both on the PEEP set by the ventilator and how completely the lungs have emptied before the next inspiration. Note that the last form of the equation shows that airway pressure (from the ventilator) must rise above $PEEP_{TOT}$ before inspiratory flow can begin.

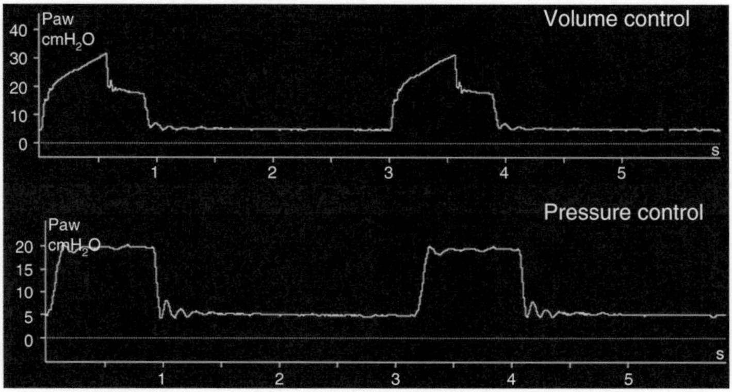

During mechanical ventilation, airway pressure depends on:

1. Lung and chest-wall compliance
2. The flow
3. AutoPEEP
4. The tidal volume
5. All the above

1.11 Equation of Motion for Spontaneously Breathing Patients

In spontaneously breathing patients, the pressure generated by the *patient's muscle* (P_{MUS}) is added to the *pressure applied by the ventilator*:

$$P_{AW} + (P_{MUS} - PEEP_{TOT}) = (\text{tidal volume / compliance}) + (\text{flow} \times \text{resistance})$$

There are two implications of this equation:

- First is that for PC modes, increasing P_{MUS} does not affect P_{AW} (because this is preset), but it increases volume and flow (i.e., it deforms the volume and flow curves). For VC modes, increasing P_{MUS} decreases P_{AW} (i.e., it deforms the pressure curve), but it does not affect volume or flow (because they are preset).
- Second, it follows that P_{MUS} must exceed $PEEP_{TOT}$ in order for P_{AW} to drop (or flow to increase) enough to trigger inspiration. Otherwise a patient-ventilator asynchrony occurs, known as an "ineffective trigger effort."

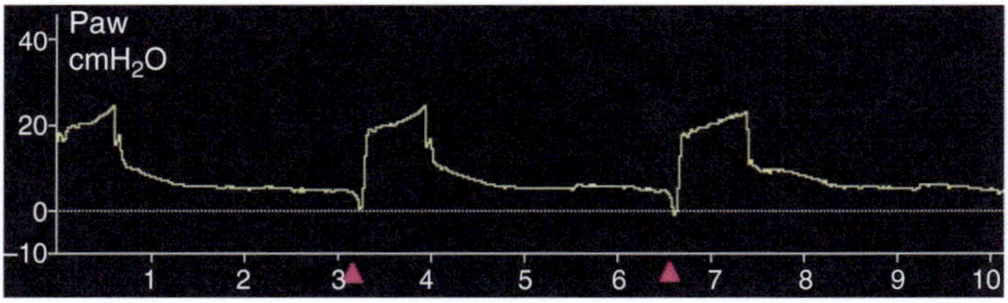

When the patient makes an inspiratory effort:

1. P_{MUS} distorts the pressure waveform in PC modes and the volume waveform in VC modes
2. P_{MUS} distorts the flow waveform in PC modes and the pressure waveform in VC modes
3. P_{MUS} must be greater than $PEEP_{TOT}$ to trigger inspiration
4. Both 2 and 3
5. None of the above

1.12 Independent and Dependent Variables

The equation of motion is the *theoretical basis for classifying modes* as "pressure control" (PC) or "volume control" (VC). Pressure control means that the left-hand side of the equation is predetermined (i.e., preset inspiratory pressure and time or inspiratory pressure is adjusted by the ventilator to be proportional to inspiratory effort) with volume and flow delivery dependent on the patient's respiratory mechanics. Hence, pressure is considered the independent variable, while volume and flow are dependent variables.

Volume control means that the right-hand side of the equation is predetermined (preset tidal volume and flow) making pressure delivery dependent on the patient's respiratory mechanics. Thus, volume and flow are considered independent variables in the equation of motion, and pressure is the dependent variable.

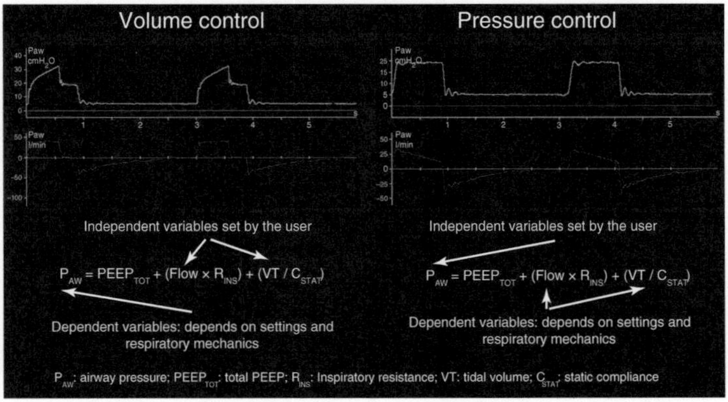

To identify the control variable:

1. A constant inspiratory pressure indicates PC
2. A constant inspiratory flow indicates VC
3. If tidal volume and flow are both preset, this indicates VC
4. If inspiratory pressure is preset, this indicates PC
5. All of the above

1.13 Which Curves Should Be Monitored During Inspiration?

The independent-variable curve provides information on the control variable of the ventilator. The dependent-variable curve indicates the response of the respiratory system. Thus, for monitoring the patient, the essential information is obtained by looking at the *dependent-variable curve.*

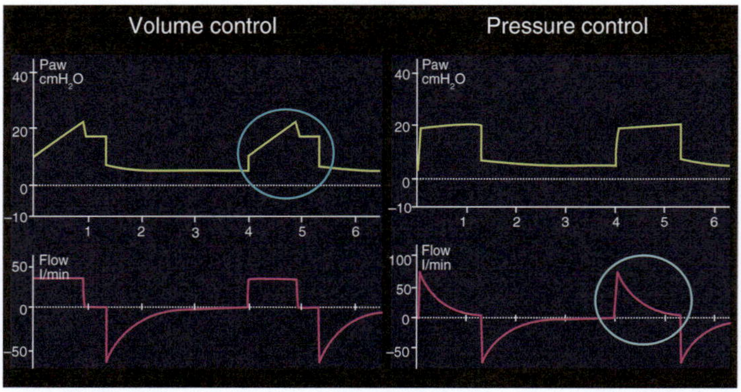

The dependent variable is:

1. The pressure curve in VC modes
2. The pressure curve in PC modes
3. The flow curve in PC modes
4. Both 1 and 3
5. The flow curve in VC modes

1.14 Compliance

Respiratory-system compliance is the ratio between a *change in volume and the associated change in pressure*. Elastance is the reciprocal of compliance ($E_{RS} = 1/C_{RS}$). Respiratory-system elastance is the sum of lung elastance and chest-wall elastance.

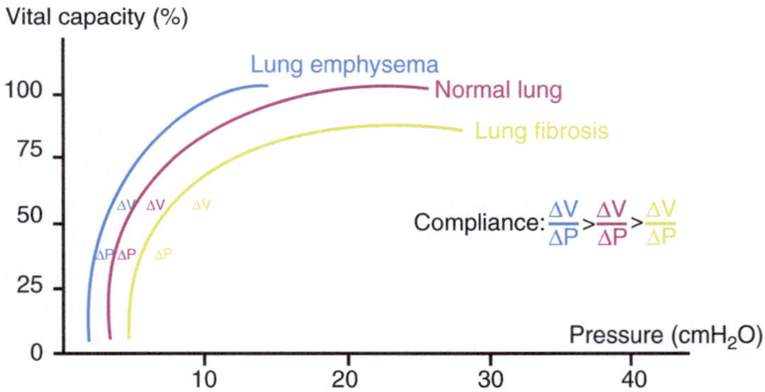

Compliance is expressed in:

1. cm H_2O/L
2. mL/cm H_2O
3. hPa
4. L/min
5. cm H_2O/L/s

1.15 Static and Dynamic Compliance

Static compliance is the ratio of tidal volume to driving pressure and represents the elasticity of the respiratory system. It is calculated as the ratio of volume change to pressure change ($\Delta V/\Delta P$) between two points in time when flow throughout the respiratory system is zero (e.g., during an inspiratory pause maneuver): $C_{STAT} = V_T/(P_{PLAT} - PEEP_{TOT})$.

Dynamic compliance is the estimation of C_{STAT} during dynamic conditions (i.e., during active inspiration without the use of an inspiratory hold). Thus, it is the ratio of volume change to pressure change between two points in time when flow at the airway opening is zero. This is accomplished by fitting multiple data points (e.g., pressure, volume, and flow measured every 20 ms) to the equation of motion and then solving for compliance. For the single-compartment model of the respiratory system, $C_{STAT} = C_{DYN}$ and is independent of respiratory rate. For a multiple-compartment model of the lungs, as the distribution of resistance and compliance become less homogeneous, C_{STAT} becomes greater than C_{DYN} because flow persists among lung units with different mechanical properties (pendelluft) and this flow increases ΔP for the same ΔV. In this case, C_{DYN} decreases as respiratory rate increases. Unfortunately, some authors have propagated an old idea that dynamic compliance can be calculated using peak inspiratory pressure (i.e., P_{PEAK} rather than P_{PLAT}): $C_{DYN} = V_T/(P_{PEAK} - PEEP)$. Because P_{PEAK} is a function of both R and C, clearly this metric is not a form of "compliance." This outdated definition of C_{DYN} is both clinically irrelevant and theoretically misleading.

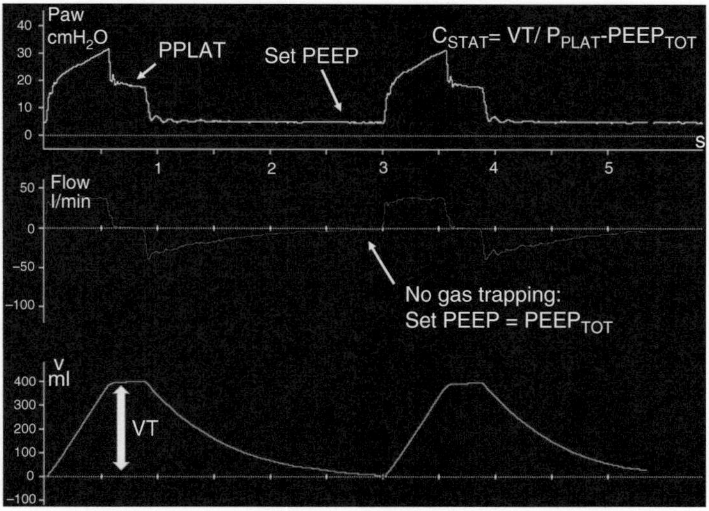

Static compliance is:

1. ΔV/ΔP
2. ΔP/ΔV
3. Not affected by gas trapping
4. Calculated using peak inspiratory pressure
5. Increased when respiratory rate increases

1.16 Resistance

Airway resistance is the ratio between the pressure driving a given flow, i.e., transairway pressure, and the resulting flow rate.

In passive patients ventilated in VC modes with a square flow waveform, airway resistance including the resistance of the endotracheal tube can be calculated as $(P_{PEAK} - P_{PLAT})$/flow.

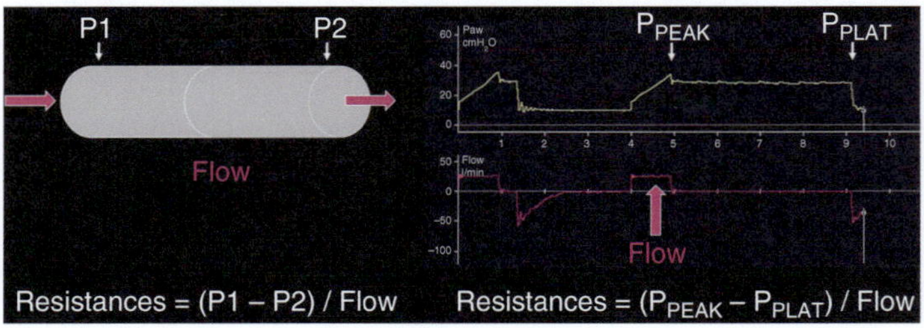

Inspiratory resistance depends on:

1. Inspiratory flow
2. The caliber of the endotracheal tube
3. The density of the gas
4. The use of HME or heated humidification
5. All of the above

1.17 Dynamic Respiratory Mechanics: Time Constant

When a step change in pressure is applied to the respiratory system, the change in volume (and flow and alveolar pressure) follows an exponential curve that is initially fast, but slows down progressively as it reaches a new equilibrium. The *speed of the volume change* is described by the time constant, which has the dimension of time. Mathematically, one time constant is equal to the product of resistance and compliance and describes the time needed to increase or decrease volume by 63% of the total volume change.

The time constant can be calculated during inspiration or expiration. Because the time constant represents the response to a step change (i.e., a square pressure waveform), the inspiratory time constant (RC_{INSP}) will be inaccurate to the extent that rise time is not zero (and it never is for a mechanical system). The expiratory time constant (RC_{EXP}) is almost completely dependent from the patient (assuming passive expiration so that $P_{MUS} = 0$) and independent of settings, to the extent that the pressure drops instantaneously to PEEP (which is never quite true because of resistance in the ventilator's expiratory circuit). RC_{EXP} is therefore the preferred metric of the patient's dynamic respiratory mechanics, provided there is no active expiratory effort.

The time constant is important because it determines the amount of inspiratory time required for complete tidal volume delivery during PC modes.

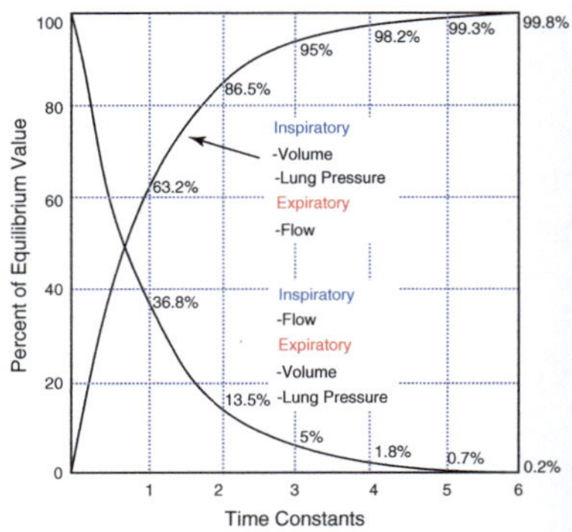

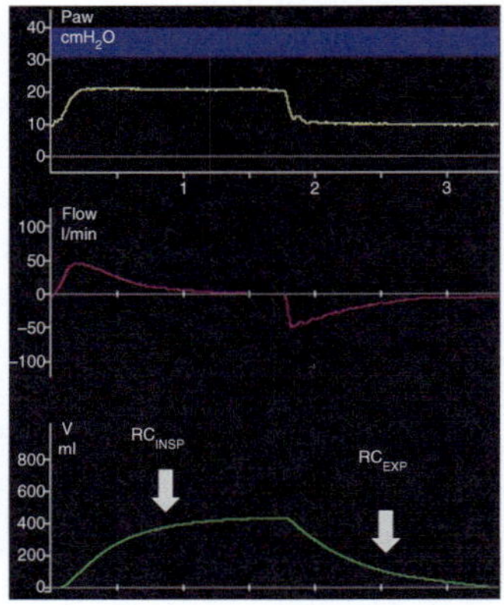

In terms of the time constant:

1. The inspiratory and expiratory time constants are equal
2. Three expiratory time constants equal the time required to exhale 95% of the tidal volume
3. The time constant depends primarily on compliance
4. A short time constant means increased resistance
5. The inspiratory time constant depends on the inspiratory time

1.18 Expiratory Time Constant

Some ventilators provide a measurement of the RC_{EXP} in all ventilation modes, including NIV. This measurement is accurate if there is no active expiratory effort and no leakage.

For an intubated patient with normal lungs, the RC_{EXP} is usually between 0.5 and 0.7 s.

A decrease in the lung and/or the chest-wall compliance (e.g., ARDS) is associated with a short RC_{EXP} (< 0.5 s).

An increase in airway and/or endotracheal tube resistance (e.g., COPD) is associated with a long RC_{EXP} (> 0.7 s).

The expiratory time constant determines the time required for complete exhalation during any mode. Thus, if expiratory time is set less than five time constants, gas trapping will occur and $PEEP_{TOT}$ increases above set PEEP (i.e., autoPEEP >0).

	Normal lung	**ARDS**	**COPD**
C_{STAT} (ml/cm H_2O)	45–65	< 45	50–80
R_{INS} (cm H_2O s/l)	10–15	10–15	16–33
RC_{EXP} (s)	0.5–0.7	< 0.5	> 0.7

The expiratory time constant:

1. Is accurate only in passive patients
2. Reflects the disease state of the respiratory system
3. Is expressed in seconds
4. Is slightly different in intubated patients and those receiving NIV
5. All of the above

1.19 Clinical Application of the Expiratory Time Constant

A normal RC_{EXP} (0.5–0.7 s) means a normal lung or a mixed condition (COPD + ARDS).

A short RC_{EXP} (< 0.5 s) means there is decreased compliance due to the lung and/or the chest wall: ARDS, lung fibrosis, atelectasis, kyphoscoliosis, increased abdominal pressure, etc.

A long RC_{EXP} (> 0.7 s) means there are increased resistances due to the patient and/or the endotracheal tube: COPD, asthma, bronchospasm, endotracheal tube obstruction, etc.

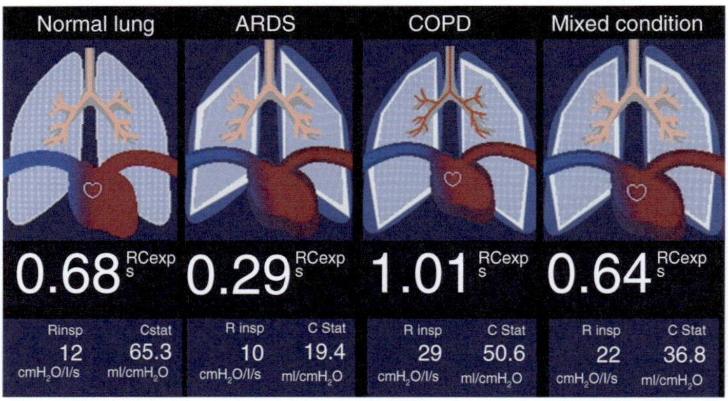

The expiratory time constant:

1. Is approximately 0.6 s in normal-lung patients
2. Is approximately 0.3 s in the case of ARDS
3. Is long in COPD and asthmatic patients
4. Can be normal in the case of a mixed-disease condition
5. All of the above

1.20 Rationale Behind Curve Analysis

Airway flow and pressure curves display the *complex interaction* between the ventilator settings and the patient's respiratory mechanics. In fact, pressure, volume, and flow curves displayed by the ventilator are nothing more than graphical representations of the equation of motion.

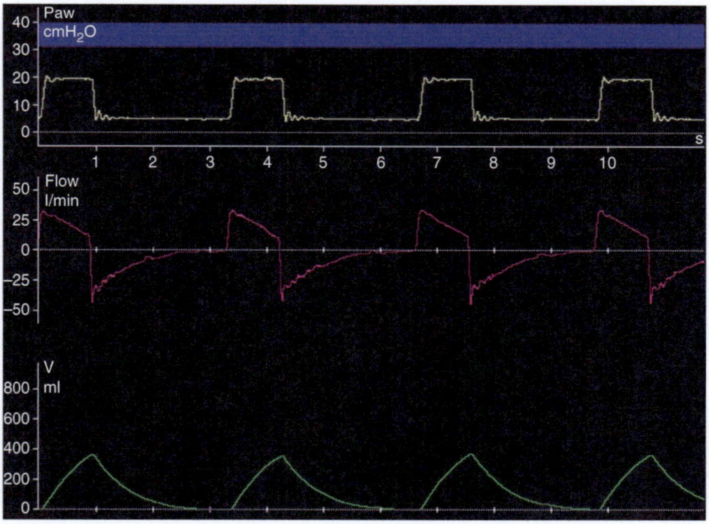

An analysis of the curves is used to:

1. Assess the patient's respiratory mechanics
2. Optimize the ventilator settings
3. Both 1 and 2
4. Predict the gas exchange
5. Learn the geography

Responses

1.1 4

1.2 4

1.3 1

1.4 2: Some ventilators measure airway pressure directly at proximal airways, between the Y piece and the endotracheal tube. Others measure it remotely at the inspiratory compartment (between the inspiratory valve and the inspiratory gas outlet) and at the expiratory compartment (between the expiratory gas inlet and the expiratory valve). Then, proximal airway pressure is calculated taking into account the breathing circuit resistances

1.5 4

1.6 3

1.7 3

1.8 5

1.9 5

1.10 5: AutoPEEP if any is part of total PEEP. Total PEEP = external PEEP + autoPEEP

1.11 4

1.12 5

1.13 4

1.14 2

1.15 1

1.16 5

1.17 2: Inspiratory and expiratory time constant are not equal because airway resistances are usually lower during inspiration as compared to expiration. Thus, inspiratory time constant is shorter than expiratory time constant

Time constant	Change in volume (% of total change)
1	63%
2	86.5%
3	95%
4	98%
5	99%

1.18 5: RC_{EXP} is slightly different in intubated and NIV patients because of the ET resistance

1.19 5

1.20 3

Suggested Readings

Arnal JM, Garnero A, et al. Parameters for simulation of adult subjects during mechanical ventilation. Respir Care 2017; in press.

Brunner JX, Laubsher T, et al. Simple method to measure total expiratory time constant based on passive expiratory flow-volume curve. Crit Care Med. 1995;23:1117–22.

Chatburn RL, Mireles-Cabodevila E. Design and function of mechanical ventilators. In: Web A, Angus DC, Finfer S, Gattinoni L, Singer M, editors. Oxford textbook of critical care. 2nd ed. Oxford: Oxford University Press; 2016. chapt 92.

Chatburn RL, El-Khatib M, et al. A taxonomy for mechanical ventilation: 10 fundamental maxims. Respir Care. 2014;59:1747–63.

D'Angelo E, Calderini E, et al. Respiratory mechanics in anesthetized paralyzed humans: effects of flow, volume, and time. J Appl Physiol. 1989;67:2556–64.

Dhand R. Ventilator graphics and respiratory mechanics in the patient with obstructive lung disease. Respir Care. 2005;50:246–61.

Gattinoni L, Chiumello D, et al. Bench-to-bedside review: chest wall elastance in acute lung injury/acute respiratory distress syndrome patients. Crit Care. 2004;8:350–5.

Georgopoulos D, Prinianakis G, et al. Bedside waveforms interpretation as a tool to identify patient-ventilator asynchronies. Intensive Care Med. 2006;32:34–47.

Hess DR. Respiratory mechanics in mechanically ventilated patients. Respir Care. 2014;59:1773–94.

Hess DR, Bigatello LM. The chest wall in acute lung injury/acute respiratory distress syndrome. Curr Opin Crit Care. 2008;14:94–102.

Iotti G, Braschi A. Measurement of respiratory mechanics during mechanical ventilation. Rhäzüns, Switzerland: Hamilton Medical Scientific Library; 1999.

Iotti GA, Braschi A, et al. Respiratory mechanics by least squares fitting in mechanically ventilated patients: applications during paralysis and during pressure support ventilation. Intensive Care Med. 1995;21:406–13.

Lourens MS, Van Den Berg B, et al. Expiratory time constants in mechanically ventilated patients with and without COPD. Intensive Care Med. 2000;26:1612–8.

Nilsestuen JO, Hargett KD. Using ventilator graphics to identify patient-ventilator asynchrony. Respir Care. 2005;50:202–34.

Stahl CA, Möller K, et al. Dynamic versus static respiratory mechanics in acute lung injury and acute respiratory distress syndrome. Crit Care Med. 2006;34:2090–8.

Stenqvist O. Practical assessment of respiratory mechanics. Br J Anaesth. 2003;91:92–105.

Chapter 2
Controlled Modes

2.1 Volume-Controlled Modes

2.1.1 Shape of the Pressure Curve

During VC, *flow and tidal volume* are the independent variables set by the user. In the simplest case, the flow waveform is square (constant flow) during inspiration. Pressure is the dependent variable. Pressure increases during insufflation to reach a maximum at the end of inspiration. If an end-inspiratory pause is set by the user, the flow will be zero and pressure will reach a plateau (Video 2.1).

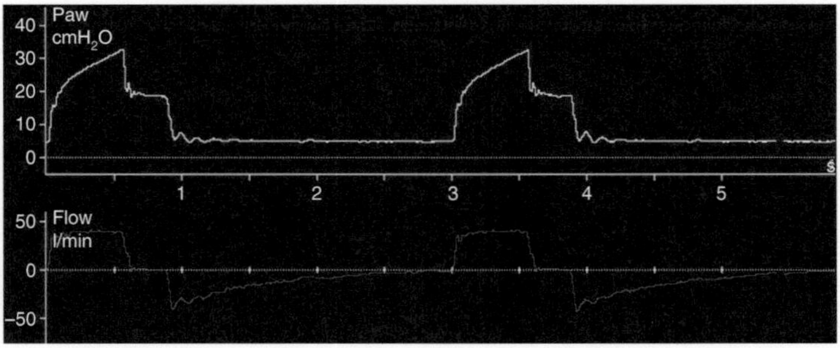

Electronic Supplementary Material The online version of this chapter (https://doi.org/10.1007/978-3-319-58655-7_2) contains supplementary material, which is available to authorized users.

J.-M. Arnal, *Monitoring Mechanical Ventilation Using Ventilator Waveforms*, https://doi.org/10.1007/978-3-319-58655-7_2

In VC modes with constant flow:

1. The flow curve provides information about respiratory mechanics
2. Pressure is the independent variable
3. Pressure reaches its maximum at the end of the inspiratory time
4. The pressure curve shows always a plateau
5. The pressure curve has a square shape

2.1.2 Flow Pattern

Different flow waveforms can be set in during VC on some ventilators:

- *Square*: Flow is constant throughout the inspiratory phase. This pattern is associated with the highest peak pressure.
- *Descending ramp*: Flow is at its maximum at the beginning of inspiration and decreases linearly during the inspiratory phase.
- *Sine*: Flow gradually increases to a maximum at mid-inspiratory time and then decreases back down to zero (Video 2.2)

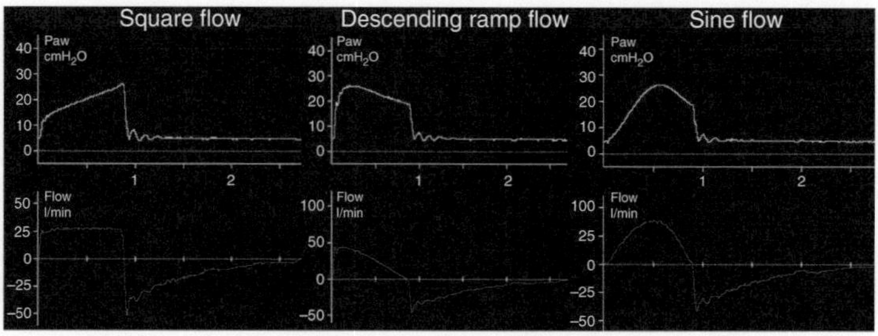

In VC, the preset flow waveform affects all these variables *except*:

1. The tidal volume delivered
2. The inspiratory time
3. The peak pressure
4. The shape of the pressure curve
5. The gas distribution within the lung

2.1.3 *Resistive Component of the Pressure Curve*

If only the resistive component of the linear one-compartment model (namely the tube) is ventilated in VC with a square flow pattern, the pressure curve will show a *square* with constant pressure throughout the inspiratory phase. The pressure will be higher if tube resistance or flow increase. Therefore, the initial rapid increase in pressure in VC is due to resistance and is reproduced at the end of inspiration by the difference between peak and plateau pressure.

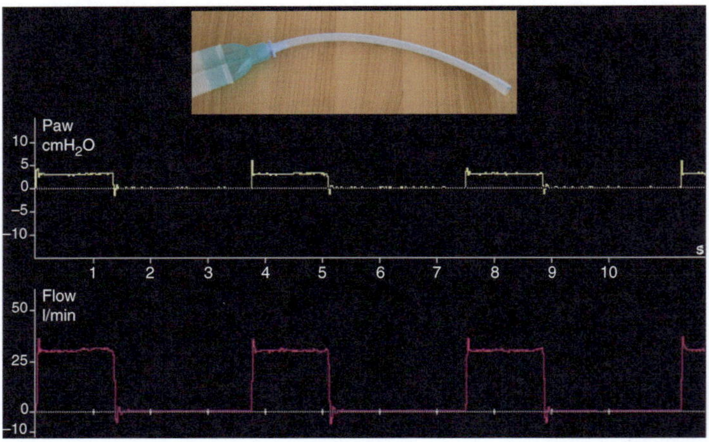

In VC, the initial increase in pressure depends on:

1. Airway resistance and flow
2. The inspiratory time
3. The size of the endotracheal tube
4. Both 1 and 3
5. Respiratory-system compliance

2.1.4 Elastic Component of the Pressure Curve

If only the elastic component of the linear one-compartment model (namely, the balloon) is ventilated in VC with a square flow waveform, the pressure curve will show a *triangle* with a gradual increase in pressure during the inspiratory phase. The slope of the pressure is proportional to respiratory-system elastance.

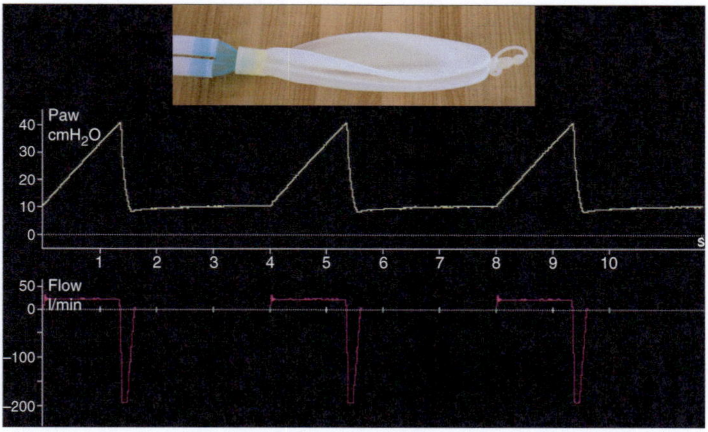

In VC, the gradual increase in pressure during inspiration:

1. Is linear at a constant flow
2. Has an exponential shape
3. Is steeper in the case of low respiratory-system compliance
4. Is steeper if V_T is increased
5. Both 1 and 3

2.1.5 The Pressure Curve for the RC Model

If both components of the model (*resistance and compliance*) are ventilated in VC with a square flow waveform, the pressure curve will show an initial rapid increase due to resistance (resistive pressure), followed by a gradual linear increase in pressure depending on compliance of the respiratory system (elastic pressure). As predicted by the equation of motion, for VC, pressure is a function of compliance, tidal volume, resistance, and flow.

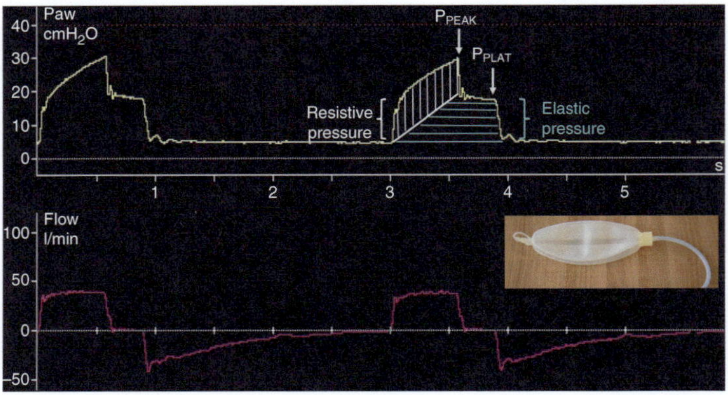

In VC, the shape of the pressure curve during inspiration is affected by:

1. Tidal volume
2. Flow
3. Resistance
4. Compliance
5. All of the above

2.1.6 *Single-Breath Analysis of Overdistension and Recruitment*

At a constant flow, the slope of the airway pressure-time curve is *proportional to elastance* (or inversely proportional to compliance). Accordingly, a pressure waveform with a constant slope suggests that compliance is constant throughout the inspiration phase, and this has been our assumption using the single-compartment model of the respiratory system. However, real respiratory systems seldom display constant compliance throughout inspiration. This is reflected in a changing slope of the pressure-time curve. Upward convexity (sometimes called concave downward) means that compliance is increasing during inspiration, suggesting tidal recruitment. Conversely, a downward convexity (also called concave upward) means that compliance is decreasing during inspiration, suggesting lung overdistension and increased risk of volutrauma.

This analysis is only accurate in passive patients ventilated in VC with gas delivered at a constant flow.

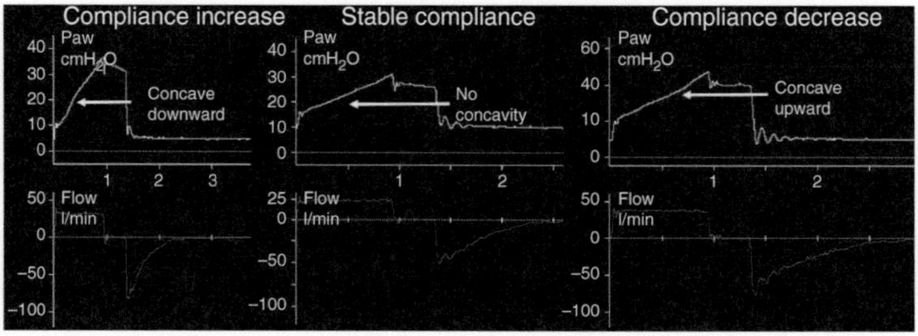

In VC, the rate of change in airway pressure:

1. Is decreasing for a normal lung
2. Suggests lung overdistension if there is upward concavity
3. May be oscillating
4. Suggests tidal recruitment if there is upward convexity
5. Should not change if PEEP is increased

2.1.7 Stress Index

The information about compliance conveyed by the pressure-time curve can be characterized using a simple mathematical model. The model is of the form

$$P_{AW} = k \times tb$$

where P_{AW} is the airway pressure, t is the time, k is a constant of proportionality (to make time equal pressure), and b is a parameter that describes the degree of concavity of the pressure-time curve. If $b = 1$, then the pressure-time curve is a straight line, there is no concavity, and compliance is constant throughout inspiration. If $b < 1$, pressure decreases with time and the pressure-time curve is concave downward because compliance increases during inspiration (recruitment). If $b > 1$, pressure increases with time and the pressure-time curve is concave upward because compliance decreases during inspiration (overdistension). The parameter b has been called the stress index. It is automatically calculated by some ventilators.

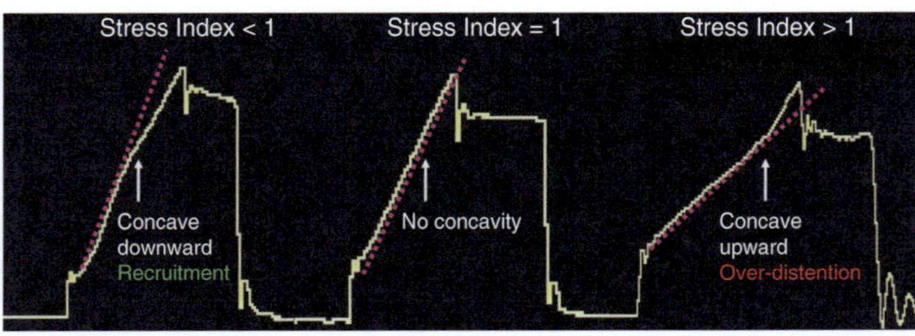

If the stress index in VC is:

1. < 1, the tidal volume could be increased
2. < 1, PEEP should be increased
3. > 1, the tidal volume should be decreased
4. > 1, PEEP should be decreased
5. All of the above

2.1.8 Peak Pressure

Peak pressure (P_{PEAK}) is the *maximum pressure* recorded during inspiration. According to the equation of motion, P_{PEAK} depends on $PEEP_{TOT}$, flow, inspiratory resistance, V_T, and respiratory-system compliance (assuming $P_{MUS} = 0$).

Therefore, any worsening of respiratory mechanics is associated with an increase in P_{PEAK}.

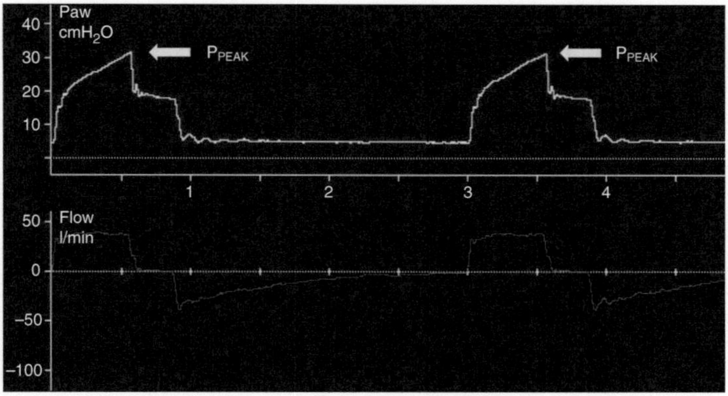

In VC, P_{PEAK} is influenced by:

1. PEEP
2. Lung compliance
3. The respiratory rate
4. Resistance
5. All of the above

2.1.9 Plateau Pressure

Plateau pressure (P_{PLAT}) is an assessment of the *alveolar pressure at the end of inspiration*. P_{PLAT} is measured by closing the ventilator valves at the end of inspiration. This can be done at each breath by setting an end-inspiratory pause or intermittently by manually performing an end-inspiratory occlusion. Due to the fact that there is no more flow (in or out of the lungs), the pressure measured at the airway opening is in equilibrium with the alveolar pressure (assuming $P_{MUS} = 0$).

According to the equation of motion, P_{PLAT} depends on $PEEP_{TOT}$, V_T, and respiratory-system compliance.

The pressure drop between P_{PEAK} and P_{PLAT} is called transairway pressure and represents the resistive pressure.

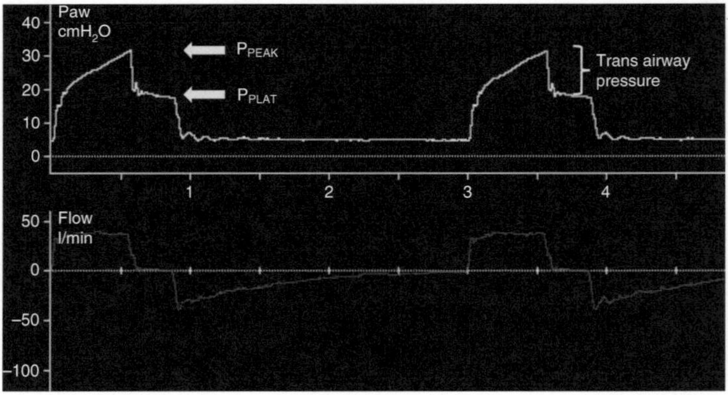

In VC, P_{PLAT} is influenced by all these variables *except*:

1. The flow waveform
2. The chest-wall compliance
3. The lung compliance
4. The tidal volume
5. The PEEP

2.1.10 *End-Inspiratory Occlusion*

In patients with normal lungs, an end-inspiratory occlusion of at least 0.5 s allows for an accurate measurement of P_{PLAT}. However, in patients with a diseased lung associated with lung inhomogeneity, a longer end-inspiratory occlusion of up to 5 s is required to reach a plateau. This long end-inspiratory occlusion must be performed manually (Video 2.3).

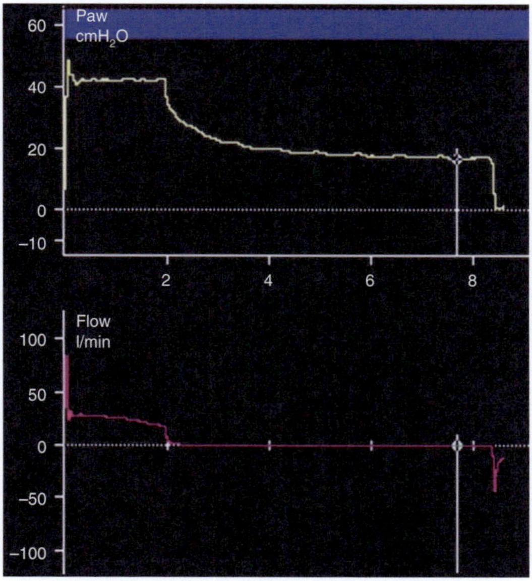

In VC, P_{PLAT} is measured using:

1. A short end-inspiratory pause for normal-lung patients
2. A manual 5-second end-inspiratory occlusion in COPD patients
3. A short end-inspiratory pause in COPD patients
4. A short end-inspiratory occlusion in ARDS patients
5. All but 3

2.1.11 End-Inspiratory Occlusion with Leakage

The plateau pressure will be *unstable* in the case of leakage from the ventilator circuit or a bronchopleural fistula or leak around the endotracheal tube (e.g., cuffless tubes used in children). Using this plateau pressure to calculate compliance or resistance will result in inaccurate respiratory mechanics values.

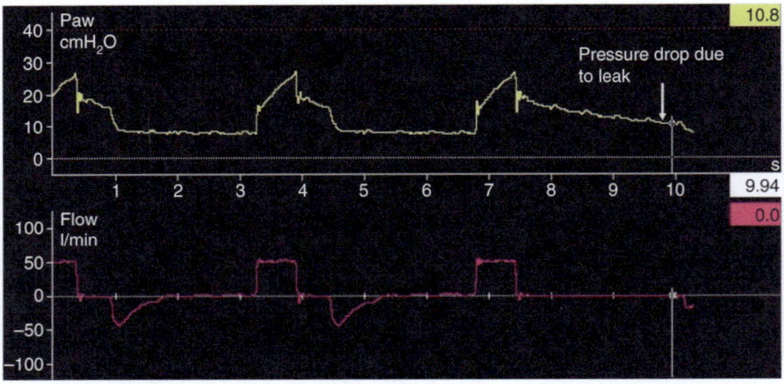

A decreasing plateau pressure during an end-inspiratory occlusion can be caused by:

1. Leakage from the ventilator circuit
2. A bronchopleural fistula
3. An underinflated endotracheal tube cuff
4. Nebulization during the occlusion
5. All but 4

2.1.12 End-Inspiratory Occlusion with Active Effort

The plateau pressure will be *unstable* with a negative pressure swing in the case of an active inspiratory effort and a positive pressure swing in case of an active expiratory effort. In such cases, measuring the plateau pressure is not recommended because the patient is not completely relaxed.

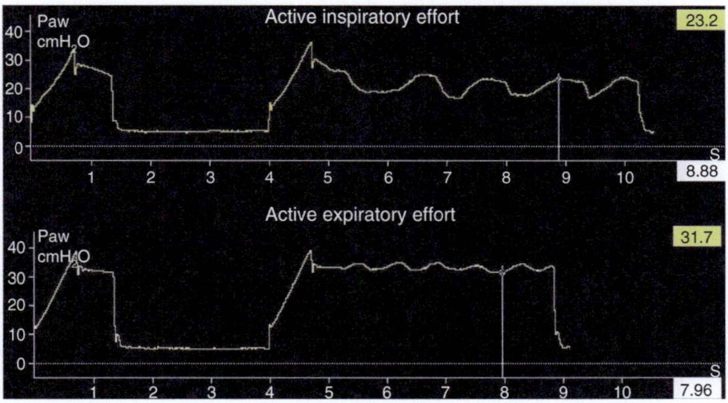

When performing an end-inspiratory occlusion, all are true *except*:

1. The plateau pressure is stable if the patient is fully relaxed and there is no leak
2. A negative pressure swing occurs in the case of an inspiratory effort
3. The plateau pressure can be measured between two swings
4. A positive pressure swing occurs in the case of an expiratory effort
5. A gradual decrease of pressure indicates a leak

2.1.13 Ascending Pressure During an End-Inspiratory Occlusion

In the case of continuous insufflation of additional gas through the ventilator circuit (e.g., inhaled nitric oxide) or continuous nebulization, the plateau pressure will *increase* progressively during an end-inspiratory occlusion. These systems should therefore be turned off during measurement.

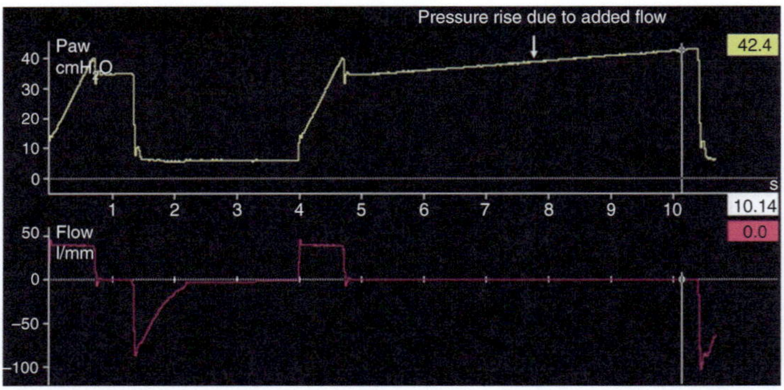

To measure plateau pressure correctly by means of an end-inspiratory occlusion:

1. There should be no leaks from the circuit
2. The plateau pressure should be stable
3. The patient should be completely relaxed
4. Additional gas (e.g., nebulizer) should be turned off temporarily
5. All of the above

2.1.14 Additional Resistance

An end-inspiratory occlusion produces an immediate drop in peak airway pressure (P_{PEAK}) down to a lower initial pressure (P_1). Then pressure continues to decline gradually—even after the ventilator valves are closed—to reach a plateau after 3–5 s (P_{PLAT}) depending on lung mechanics. Maximum resistance, ($P_{PEAK}-P_{PLAT}$)/flow, is then partitioned into minimum resistance, ($P_{PEAK}-P_1$)/flow, and additional resistance, (P_1-P_{PLAT})/flow. Minimum resistance represents the flow resistance of the airways and the endotracheal tube. Additional resistance represents the viscoelastic behavior or stress relaxation of the pulmonary tissues and decay of flow (pendelluft) among lung units with different time constants. Time-constant inequalities induce pendelluft from regions with short time constants to regions with long time constants.

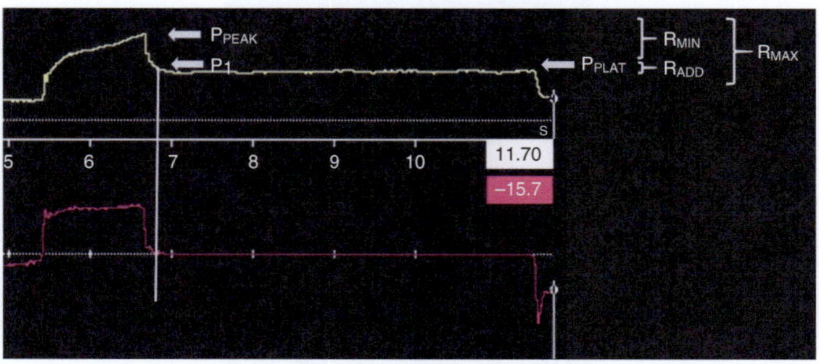

During an end-inspiratory occlusion, airway pressure:

1. Rapidly drops to plateau pressure
2. Is stable as soon as the ventilator valves are closed
3. Drops initially due to airway and ET flow resistance
4. Decreases gradually after closure of the ventilator valves to reach a plateau
5. Both 3 and 4

2.1.15 Increased Peak Pressure

According to the equation of motion, an increase in P_{PEAK} can be caused by an *increase in resistance or $PEEP_{TOT}$*, a decrease in compliance, or a combination of both. To distinguish between increased resistance and decreased compliance, the first step is to perform an end-inspiratory occlusion to measure P_{PLAT}. If P_{PLAT} has not changed, the increase in P_{PEAK} was due to an increase in resistance. If P_{PLAT} is higher, the change in P_{PLAT} resulted either from an increase in total PEEP or a decrease in compliance. Subsequently, an end-expiratory occlusion should be performed to measure total PEEP.

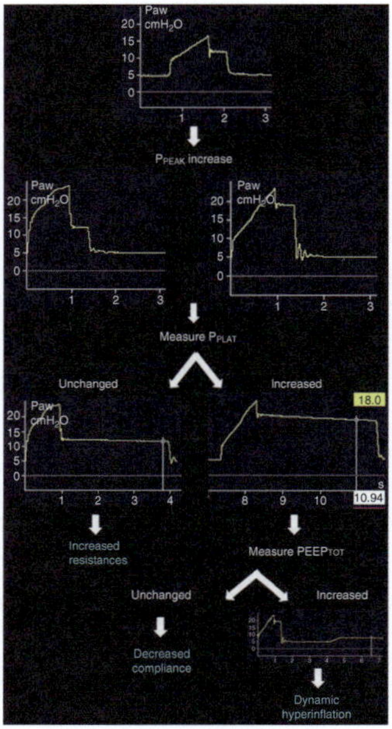

Which of the following will not activate a high pressure alarm during VC:

1. Excessive secretions in the endotracheal tube
2. A pulmonary embolism
3. Dynamic hyperinflation
4. A pneumothorax
5. A bronchospasm

2.1.16 Mean Airway Pressure

The mean airway pressure is the *average pressure over a ventilatory cycle* (one inspiration and one expiration). Graphically, it is represented by the area below the pressure-time curve divided by the ventilatory period (inspiratory time plus expiratory time). Numerically, it can be calculated by the ventilator as the average of many pressure samples (e.g., one every 20 ms) taken over the ventilatory period. Mean airway pressure is important clinically because within reasonable limits, PaO_2 is proportional to mean airway pressure. On the other hand, cardiac output may be inversely proportional to mean airway pressure.

Anything that increases airway pressure (see equation of motion) or increases the I:E ratio (increasing inspiratory time or decreasing expiratory time) increases mean airway pressure.

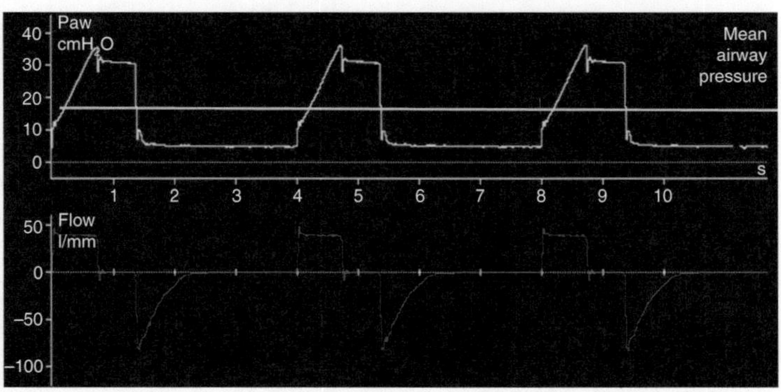

Which of the following statements is false about mean airway pressure?

1. It is the area below the pressure curve during a full breath
2. It is increased when PEEP is increased
3. It decreases in PC when inspiratory time is decreased
4. It increases with the use of an inspiratory hold in VC
5. It increases if compliance decreases

2.1.17 Driving Pressure

Driving pressure, ΔP, (more accurately, tidal pressure) is the pressure required to overcome elastic force during tidal inflation of the respiratory system. Driving pressure is calculated as

$$\Delta P = E_{RS} \times V_T = V_T / C_{STAT} = P_{PLAT} - \mathrm{PEEP}_{TOT}$$

Driving pressure is *one metric of the strain* applied to the respiratory system and the risk of volutrauma. Increased ΔP is associated with worse clinical outcomes in ARDS, postsurgical, and normal-lung patients (Video 2.4).

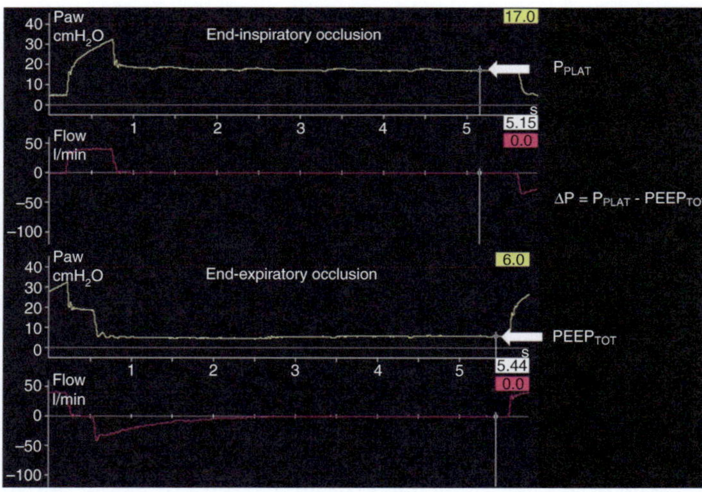

Driving pressure is increased when:

1. Tidal volume increases
2. Resistance increases
3. PEEP decreases
4. Compliance increases
5. Flow increases

2.2 Pressure-Controlled Mode

2.2.1 Flow Curve

In PC modes, the inspiratory flow is a consequence of the ventilator's attempt to maintain a preset pressure waveform. Flow has a *special shape* with a rapid increase in flow initially, followed by an exponential drop. The inspiratory flow is generated by the pressure gradient between the proximal airway and the alveoli. This gradient is at its maximum at the beginning of inspiration when alveolar pressure is equal to total PEEP. Subsequently, alveolar pressure increases gradually during inflation. As a consequence, the pressure gradient decreases. If inspiratory time is long enough, inspiratory flow drops to zero when the alveolar pressure is equal to the proximal airway pressure (Video 2.5).

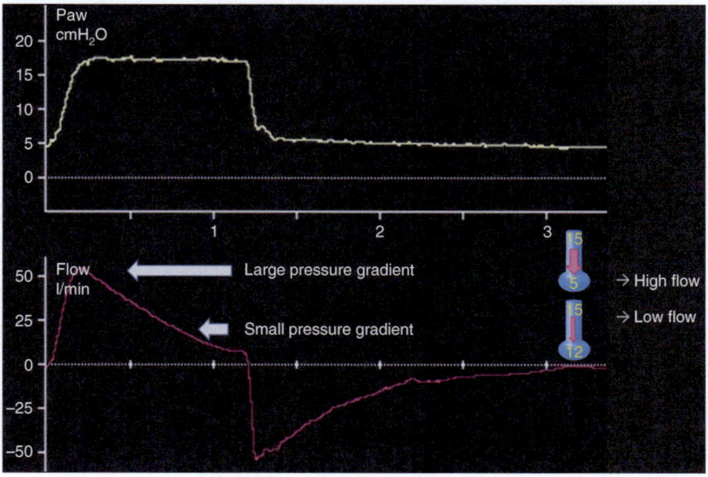

In PC, inspiratory flow:

1. Has a square shape
2. Has a shape that can be selected by the clinician
3. Is driven by the pressure gradient
4. Is at its maximum at the end of inflation
5. Never reaches zero flow

2.2.2 Peak Inspiratory Flow

Peak inspiratory flow depends on the two factors (the pressure gradient driving flow and inspiratory resistance):

$$\text{Peak flow} = \left(\text{set } P_{\text{PEAK}} - \text{PEEP}_{\text{TOT}}\right) / R_{\text{INSP}}$$

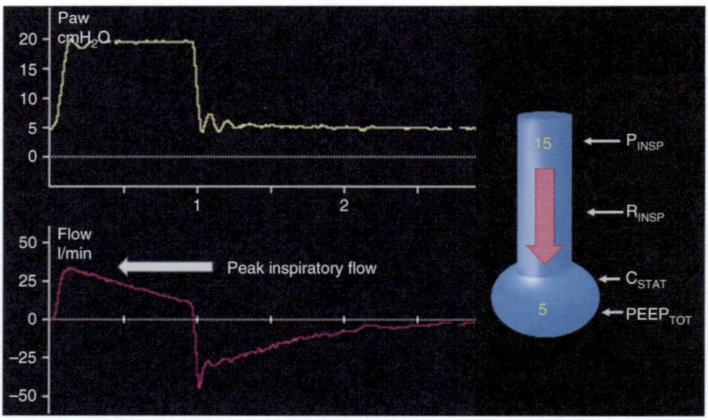

Peak inspiratory flow decreases when:

1. Intrinsic PEEP increases
2. Set inspiratory pressure increases
3. Elastance decreases
4. Resistance decreases
5. Driving pressure increases

2.2.3 Peak Inspiratory Flow Overshoot

Flow spikes on inspiration are sometimes seen in patients with high respiratory-system impedance (generally high resistance and high compliance, as in COPD). In this case, the respiratory system is acting like a two-compartment model, with one compartment (represented by the compliance of the airways and ventilator circuit) filling or emptying fast and the other (the lungs) emptying slower. During inspiration, the flow may peak initially as the airways fill with a relatively small volume and then decrease abruptly, indicating that the delay in the compensation of the pressure control algorithm in responding to the fact that not much flow is required thereafter to maintain the set pressure (essentially an overshoot error).

After the initial spike of flow, the inspiratory flow remains almost constant because most of the set pressure is being generated by the pressure drop across the high resistance and relatively little backpressure is generated by the high compliance.

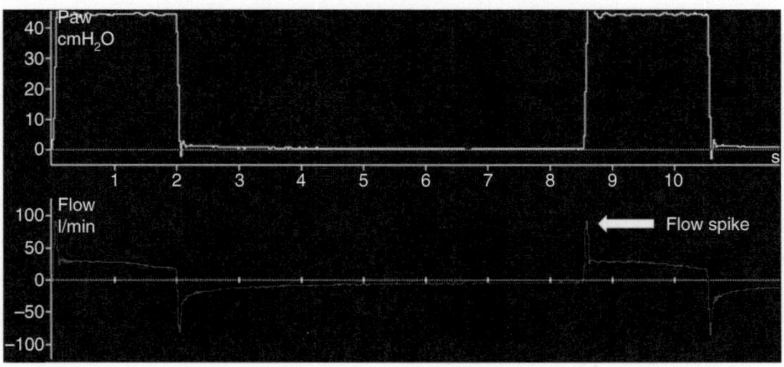

Peak inspiratory flow demonstrates a spike at the onset of inspiration in the case of:

1. Decreased compliance
2. Severe obstructive lung disease
3. High inspiratory pressure
4. Dynamic hyperinflation
5. A short inspiratory time

2.2.4 Shape of Flow Curve

Following the initial peak, the flow drops exponentially. The dynamics of the drop in flow depend on the *inspiratory time constant* (RC_{INSP}). The inspiratory time constant is the product of static compliance and inspiratory resistance. Therefore, if the time constant is short (low compliance and/or resistance), the respiratory system will inflate rapidly and inspiratory flow will drop abruptly. Conversely, if the time constant is long (high compliance and/or resistance), the respiratory system will inflate slowly and flow will drop gradually.

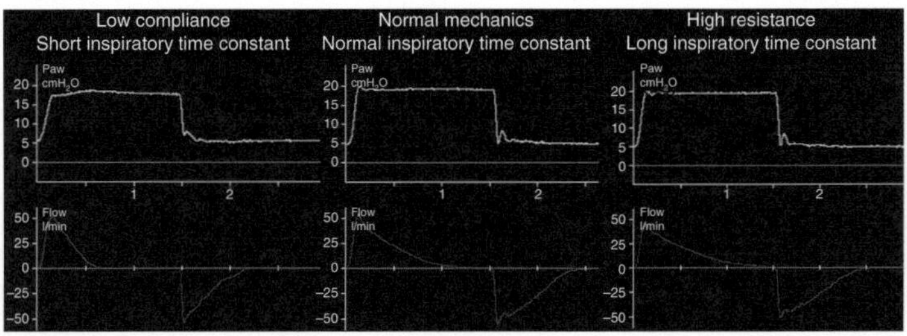

Which of these variables affect the shape of the flow curve (including peak flow and subsequent flow) and hence the associated tidal volume?

1. The time constant
2. Driving pressure
3. Resistance and compliance
4. The inspiratory time
5. All of the above

2.2.5 Inspiratory Time

A short inspiratory time may terminate inspiration before inspiratory flow reaches zero. Increasing the inspiratory time so that inspiratory flow reaches zero will result in an increase in tidal volume, without increasing the inspiratory pressure. Increasing the inspiratory time further will not change tidal volume and will provide an end-inspiratory plateau pressure (Video 2.6)

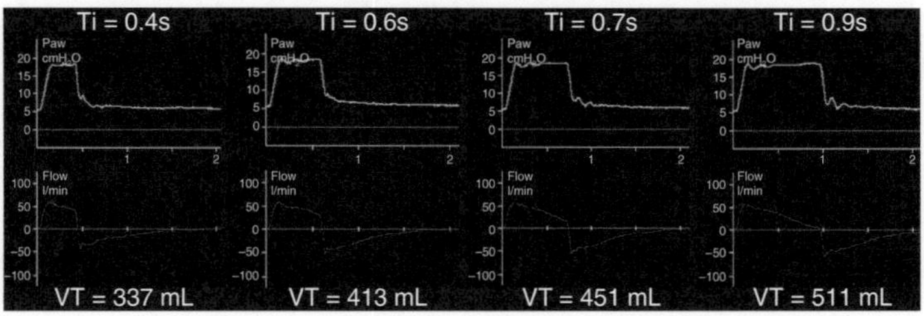

In PC, tidal volume depends on:

1. The inspiratory time
2. The driving pressure
3. The time constant
4. The intrinsic PEEP
5. All of the above

2.2.6 Inspiratory Time Optimization

For any given respiratory rate, any increase in inspiratory time is associated with a decrease in expiratory time. At some point, *dynamic hyperinflation* may occur and result in an increase in total $PEEP_{TOT}$ and a reduction in tidal volume.

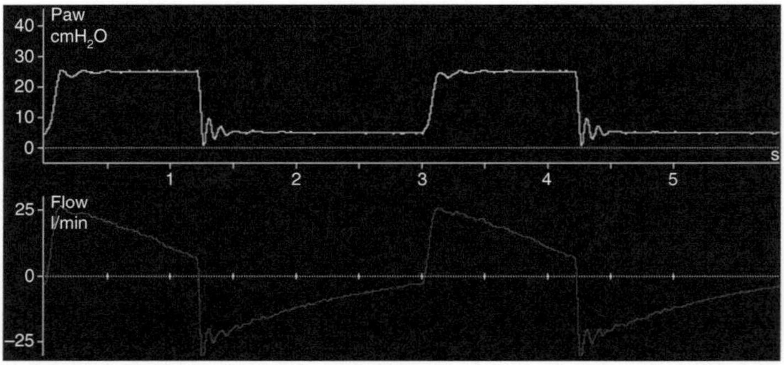

On the screenshot above, what options are available for increasing alveolar ventilation?

1. Increase the respiratory rate
2. Increase P_{INSP}
3. Increase the inspiratory time
4. Increase PEEP
5. All the above

2.2.7 Plateau Pressure

If the inspiratory *flow reaches zero at the end of inspiratory time*, it means that proximal airway pressure and alveolar pressure are equal. In this case, plateau pressure is equal to preset inspiratory pressure (P_{INSP}) above PEEP. If the inspiratory flow is still positive at the end of inspiratory time, it means that plateau pressure is lower than the preset inspiratory pressure. In such a case, an end-inspiratory occlusion is required to measure plateau pressure (Videos 2.7 and 2.8).

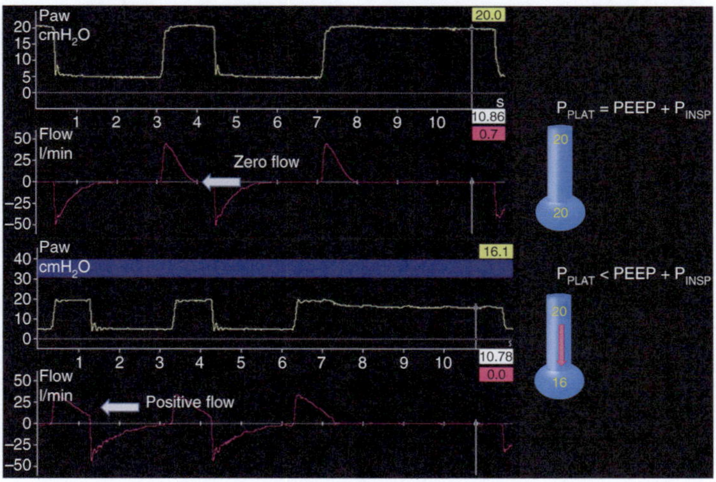

Plateau pressure in PC:

1. Is always equal to PEEP + P_{INSP}
2. Can be higher than PEEP + P_{INSP}
3. Is always lower than PEEP + P_{INSP}
4. Can be lower than PEEP + P_{INSP}
5. Can't be measured

2.2.8 Mean Airway Pressure

As in VC, the mean airway pressure is equal to the area below the pressure-time curve divided by the ventilatory period (inspiratory time plus expiratory time) and is dependent on PEEP, P_{INSP}, and the I:E ratio. The mean airway pressure is related to both *oxygenation and hemodynamic compromise* induced by mechanical ventilation.

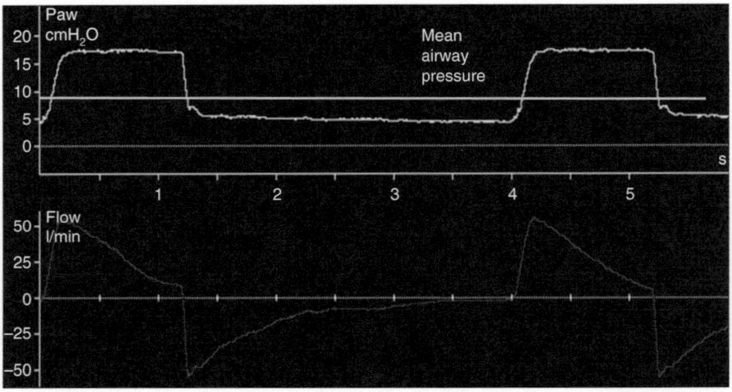

When mean airway pressure increases:

1. Cardiac output may decrease
2. Elimination of CO_2 may increase
3. Oxygenation usually improves
4. Pleural pressure increases
5. All of the above

2.2.9 Driving Pressure

Driving pressure (ΔP), or tidal pressure, is the *elastic pressure* required to inflate the respiratory system ($\Delta P = V_T/C_{STAT}$). In PC, ΔP is only equal to P_{INSP} (relative to PEEP) if inspiratory time is long enough for flow to decay to zero during inspiration and there is no autoPEEP. Therefore, ΔP is measured by performing an end-inspiratory pause (to measure P_{PLAT}) and then an end-expiratory pause (to measure P_{TOT}) for 3–5 s each (Video 2.9):

$$\Delta P = P_{PLAT} - \mathrm{PEEP}_{TOT}$$

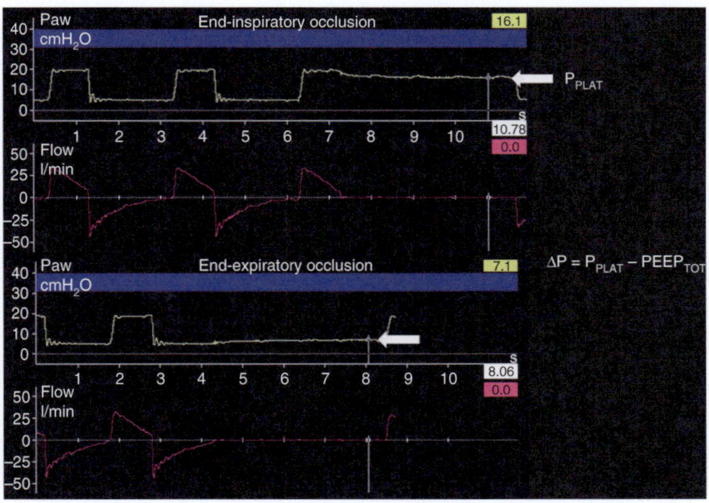

Driving pressure can be determined using all these variables *except*:

1. Tidal volume
2. autoPEEP
3. P_{PLAT}
4. The inspiratory time
5. Static compliance

Responses

2.1.1	3
2.1.2	1
2.1.3	4
2.1.4	5
2.1.5	5
2.1.6	2
2.1.7	5
2.1.8	5
2.1.9	1
2.1.10	5
2.1.11	5
2.1.12	3
2.1.13	5
2.1.14	5
2.1.15	2
2.1.16	1
2.1.17	1
2.2.1	3
2.2.2	1
2.2.3	2
2.2.4	5
2.2.5	5
2.2.6	2
2.2.7	4
2.2.8	5
2.2.9	4

Suggested Reading

Amato MB, Meade MO, et al. Driving pressure and survival in the acute respiratory distress syndrome. N Engl J Med. 2015;372:747–55.

Baedorf Kassis E, Loring SH, et al. Mortality and pulmonary mechanics in relation to respiratory system and transpulmonary driving pressures in ARDS. Intensive Care Med. 2016;42:1206–13.

Barberis L, Manno E, et al. Effect of end-inspiratory pause duration on plateau pressure in mechanically ventilated patients. Intensive Care Med. 2003;29:130–4.

Bigatello LM, Davignon KR, et al. Respiratory mechanics and ventilator waveforms in the patient with acute lung injury. Respir Care. 2005;50:235–45.

Chiumello D, Carlesso E, et al. Airway driving pressure and lung stress in ARDS patients. Crit Care. 2016;20:276.

Dhand R. Ventilator graphics and respiratory mechanics in the patient with obstructive lung disease. Respir Care. 2005;50:246–61.

Fernández-Pérez ER, Hubmayr RD. Interpretation of airway pressure waveforms. Intensive Care Med. 2006;32:658–9.

Guérin C, Papazian L, et al. Effect of driving pressure on mortality in ARDS patients during lung protective mechanical ventilation in two randomized controlled trials. Crit Care. 2016;20:384.

Iotti G, Braschi A. Measurement of respiratory mechanics during mechanical ventilation. Rhäzüns, Switzerland: Hamilton Medical Scientific Library; 1999.

Laffey JG, Bellani G, et al. Potentially modifiable factors contributing to outcome from acute respiratory distress syndrome: the LUNG SAFE study. Intensive Care Med. 2016;42:1865–76.

Marini JJ, Ravenscraft SA. Mean airway pressure: physiologic determinants and clinical importance--part 1: physiologic determinants and measurements. Crit Care Med. 1992a;20:1461–72.

Marini JJ, Ravenscraft SA. Mean airway pressure: physiologic determinants and clinical importance--part 2: clinical implications. Crit Care Med. 1992b;20:1604–16.

Neto AS, Hemmes SN, et al. Association between driving pressure and development of postoperative pulmonary complications in patients undergoing mechanical ventilation for general anaesthesia: a meta-analysis of individual patient data. Lancet Respir Med. 2016;4:272–80.

Nilsestuen JO, Hargett KD. Using ventilator graphics to identify patient-ventilator asynchrony. Respir Care. 2005;50:202–34.

Ranieri VM, Zhang H, et al. Pressure-time curve predicts minimally injurious ventilatory strategy in an isolated rat lung model. Anesthesiology. 2000;93:1320–8.

Chapter 3
Monitoring During Expiration

3.1 Which Curves Should Be Monitored During Expiration?

During expiration, airway pressure displays only the PEEP set on the ventilator (external PEEP). Therefore, an analysis of expiration relies solely on a *flow-curve analysis*, regardless of the ventilation mode.

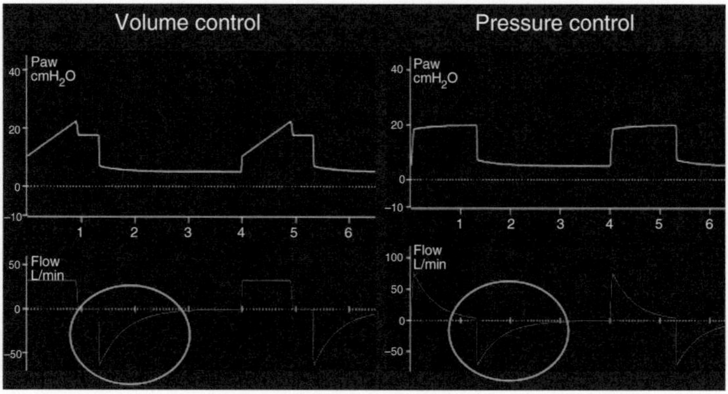

Electronic Supplementary Material The online version of this chapter (https://doi.org/10.1007/978-3-319-58655-7_3) contains supplementary material, which is available to authorized users.

J.-M. Arnal, *Monitoring Mechanical Ventilation Using Ventilator Waveforms*, https://doi.org/10.1007/978-3-319-58655-7_3

An analysis of expiration relies on:

1. The pressure curve
2. The flow curve
3. The inspiratory tidal volume
4. The cough strength
5. Whether it is performed by a saxophonist or a didgeridoo player

3.2 Normal Shape of Expiration

Normal expiration starts with a peak expiratory flow, followed by a gradual decrease in flow. At any point in time, the expiratory flow is driven by the *gradient between alveolar pressure and PEEP*. This gradient is at its maximum at the beginning of expiration and then decreases gradually.

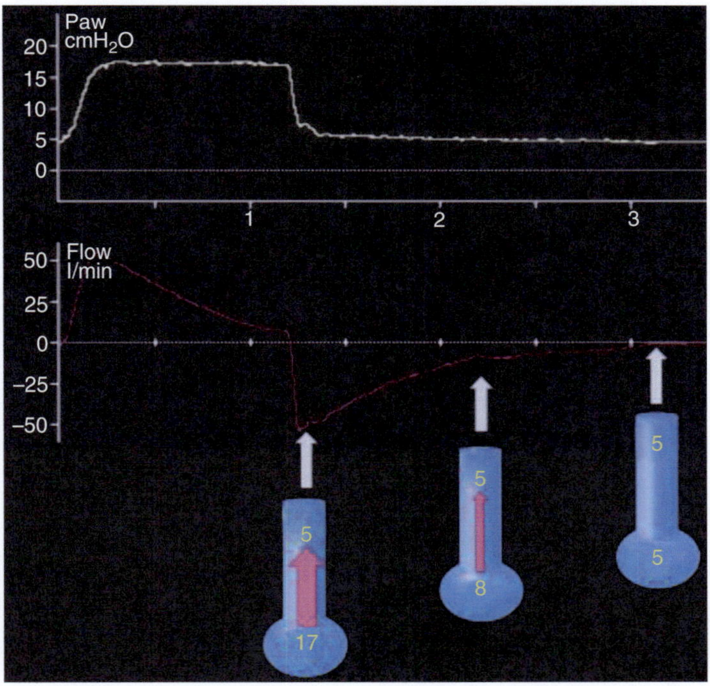

Flow during expiration:

1. May be shaped differently according to the ventilation mode
2. Starts high and decreases exponentially
3. Is square in shape
4. Depends on a pressure gradient
5. Both 2 and 4

3.3 Peak Expiratory Flow

The peak expiratory flow is driven by the *elastic recoil pressure*, which is the same as driving pressure described above. Hence:

$$\text{Peak expiratory flow} = \Delta P / R_{\text{EXP}}$$

High P_{INSP}, high tidal volume, high P_{PLAT}, and low static compliance will increase the peak expiratory flow. Conversely, high resistance and autoPEEP decrease the peak expiratory flow.

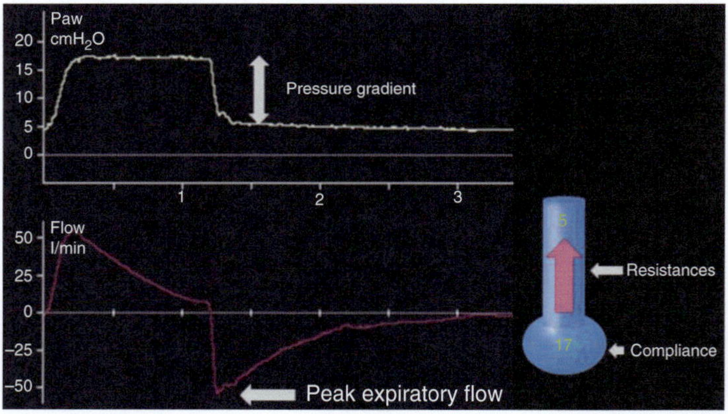

The peak expiratory flow depends on all these variables *except*:

1. The tidal volume
2. The respiratory rate
3. The end-inspiratory pause
4. Static compliance
5. The plateau pressure

3.4 Active Expiration

In mechanical ventilation, expiration is usually passive, even in spontaneously breathing patients. Active expiration may occur in the case of severe COPD (or asthma). Active expiration distorts the shape of the expiratory flow by *pushing it in the negative direction* (peak expiratory flow may also be increased depending on the timing of the expiratory effort).

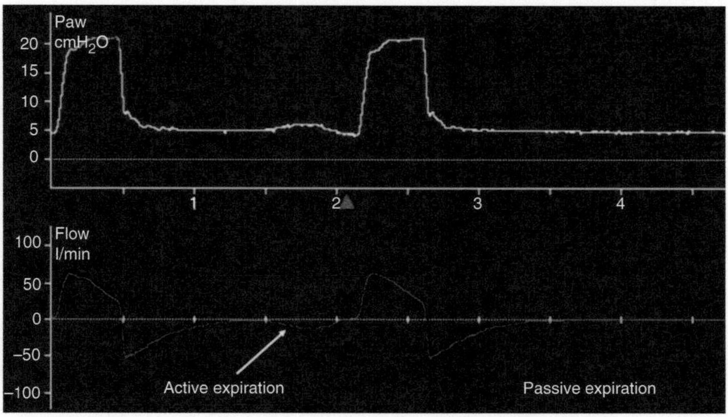

All of the following statements are true about active expiration *except*:

1. Is common in patients with COPD
2. Distorts the shape of the expiratory flow
3. May increase peak expiratory flow
4. May occur in paralyzed patients
5. Can be caused by coughing

3.5 Shape of Expiratory Flow: Normal

The shape of the expiratory flow follows an *exponential decline* down to the baseline. The dynamics of emptying the lungs depend on compliance and resistance of the respiratory system and the ventilator circuit. They are described by the expiratory time constant (RC_{EXP}), which represents the time needed to decrease the expiratory flow by 63% of the peak expiratory flow. In a normal lung, it ranges between 0.5 and 0.7 s. Two and three RC_{EXP} decrease the expiratory flow by 86% and 95% of the peak expiratory flow, respectively.

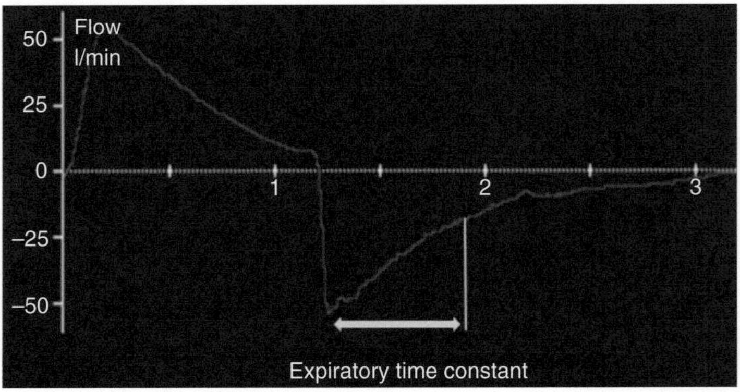

In a normal, passive patient, the expiratory flow:

1. Is shaped depending on respiratory-system mechanics
2. Lasts less than 3 s for full expiration
3. Always reaches zero before the end of the expiratory time
4. Is the same with heated humidifier and heat and moisture exchanger
5. All of the above

3.6 Shape of Expiratory Flow: Decreased Compliance

When compliance is low, elastic recoil pressure is increased. Therefore, the peak expiratory flow is increased (assuming the same tidal volume and resistance). *Expiratory time is shorter* than normal because the lung empties more quickly. The RC_{EXP} is less than 0.5 s.

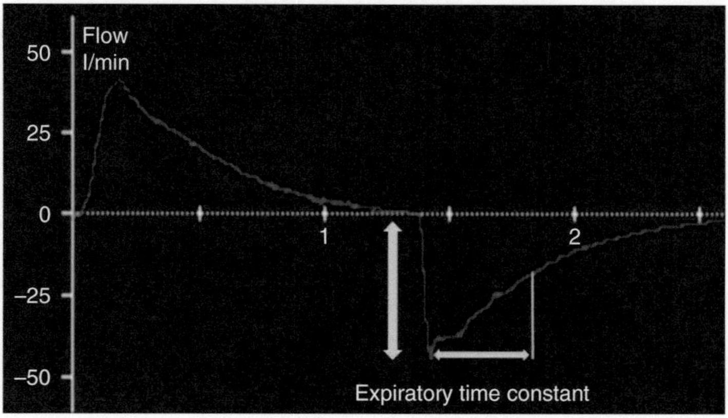

In the case of low compliance:

1. The peak expiratory flow decreases
2. Expiration takes longer
3. The expiratory flow rapidly reaches the baseline
4. RC_{EXP} is not affected
5. Full expiration lasts less than 1 s

3.7 Shape of Expiratory Flow: Increased Resistance

When resistance increases, the peak expiratory flow is lower and *expiration takes a long time* (assuming the same tidal volume and compliance). The RC_{EXP} is greater than 0.7 s.

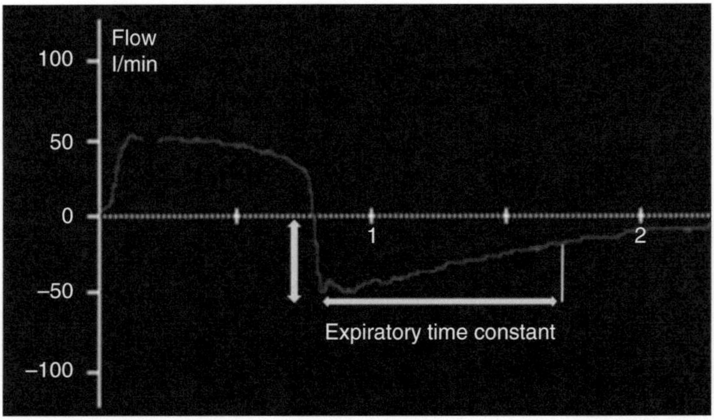

In the case of increased resistance:

1. The peak expiratory flow decreases
2. Elastic recoil pressure is decreased
3. The expiratory flow always reaches baseline
4. RC_{EXP} is decreased
5. Full expiration usually lasts <5 s

3.8 Shape of Expiratory Flow: Flow Limitation

Normally, the expiratory flow decreases in a single exponential decline. Sometimes, there may be *bi-compartmental expiration* that suggests a flow limitation. In patients with a flow limitation during expiration, an initial flow spike corresponds to a dynamic compression of gas in the central airways that is expulsed at the beginning of expiration. Thereafter, the expiratory flow decreases because flow is dependent upon the resistance and the pressure gradient from the alveoli to the choke point. Flow limitation can be shown by decreasing PEEP to zero. In a patient with normal lung, decreasing PEEP to zero should increase the expiratory flow. In contrast, in patients with expiratory flow limitation, expiratory flow does not increase when PEEP is decreased to zero. On the contrary, flow may increase when PEEP is increased if the effect of PEEP is to reduce the resistance at the choke point (Video 3.1).

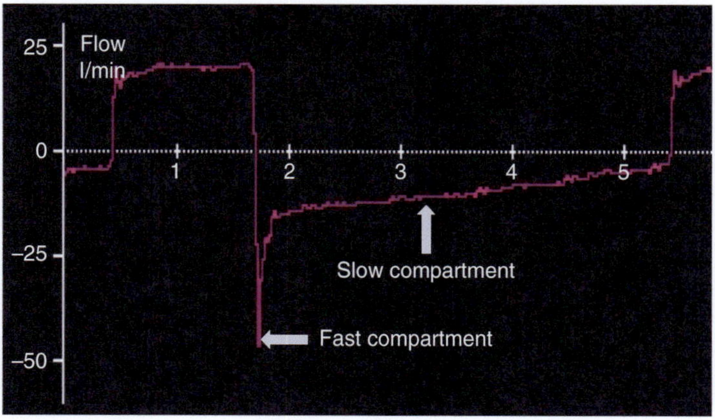

Which statement is false about expiratory flow limitation?

1. Occurs mainly in severely obstructed patients
2. Is associated with a bi-compartmental shape of expiratory flow
3. Is associated with normal expiratory time
4. Results in an increased RC_{EXP}
5. Is usually associated with dynamic hyperinflation

3.9 Secretions

The presence of *oscillations* with high frequency in the expiratory flow (and possibly pressure) waveform indicates excessive secretions or condensation in the airways or in the ventilator circuit (Video 3.2).

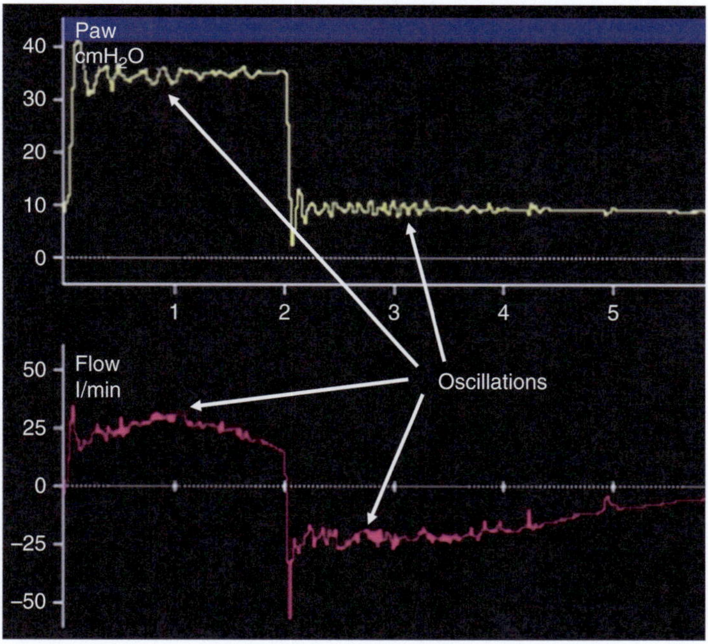

Excessive secretions in the airways can be seen as oscillations in:

1. The inspiratory pressure curve
2. The inspiratory flow curve
3. The expiratory pressure curve
4. The expiratory flow curve
5. All of the above

3.10 Bi-compartmental Expiration

Bi-compartmental expiration occurs when the lungs are *non-symmetric* with different respiratory mechanics for each lung. The fast compartment with a short expiratory time constant (low compliance and normal resistance) empties first, while the slow compartment (high compliance and increased resistance) empties later. This occurs in COPD patients with one transplanted lung. The transplanted lung is the fast compartment and the native lung the slow compartment.

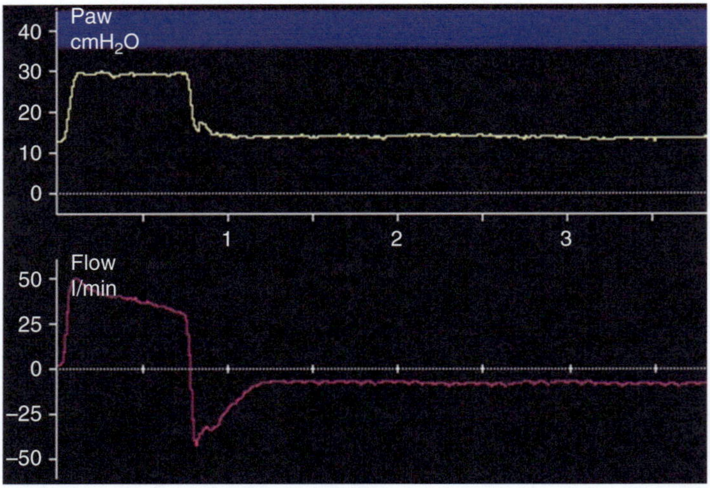

In the case of nonsymmetric lungs:

1. The expiratory flow curve is not affected
2. The compartment with the longer time constant empties first
3. The compartment with the shorter time constant empties first
4. The distribution of ventilation is unaffected
5. Only the compartment with the shorter time constant is ventilated

3.11 Tracheal Malacia

Tracheal malacia is demonstrated by *instability* of the trachea during passive expiration. The expiratory flow is restricted when the trachea collapses.

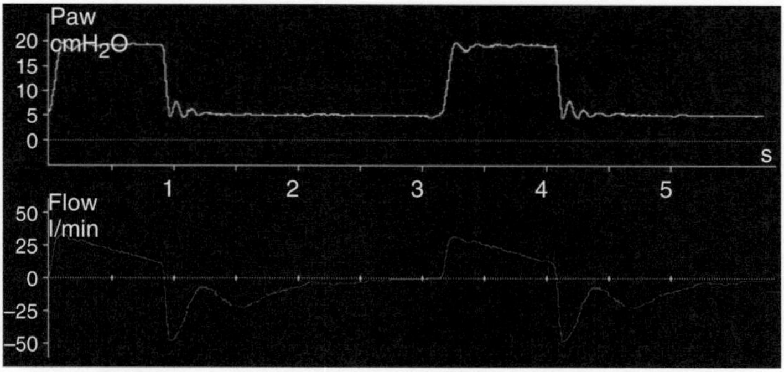

Tracheal malacia is demonstrated by:

1. Instability of the inspiratory flow
2. Instability of the expiratory flow
3. A short expiratory time constant
4. A long expiratory time constant
5. Instability of the expiratory pressure curve

3.12 End-Expiratory Flow

It is generally preferable that expiratory flow should *reach zero before the end of expiration* (an exception might be the mode called airway pressure release ventilation). Continuing flow at the end of expiration indicates dynamic hyperinflation, which induces autoPEEP. AutoPEEP reduces tidal volume during PC ventilation and may contribute to ineffective trigger efforts.

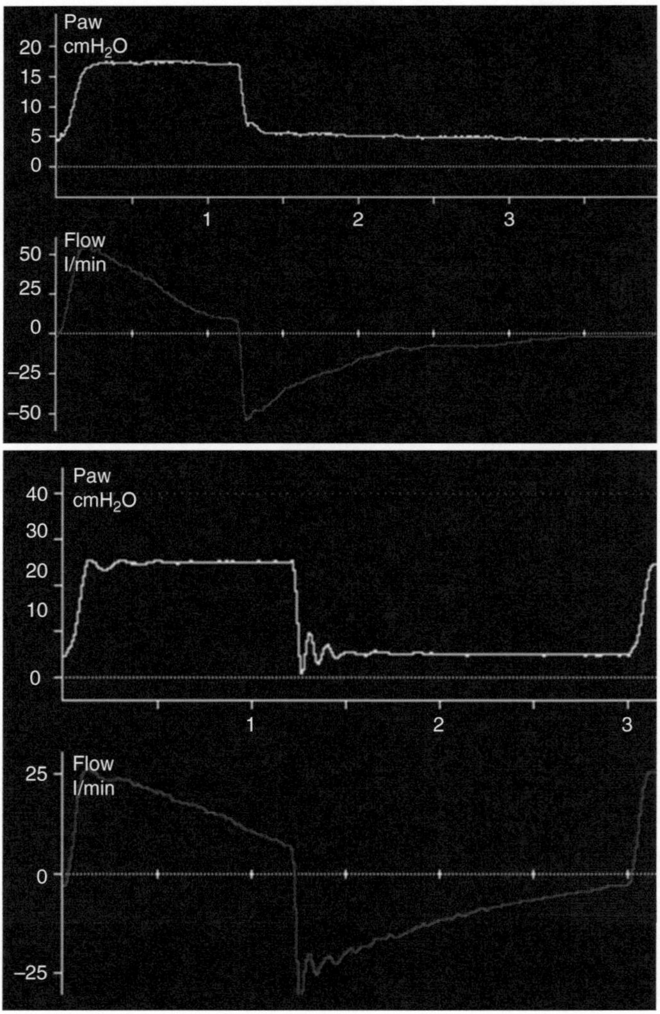

Continuing flow at the end of expiration occurs in the case of all of the following *except*:

1. High resistance
2. Low compliance
3. A short expiratory time
4. High compliance
5. An expiratory flow limitation

3.13 End-Expiratory Occlusion

An end-expiratory occlusion is used to measure *autoPEEP*. Ventilator valves are closed at the end of expiration, and pressure in the lungs equilibrates with the pressure in the ventilator circuit. Thus, the pressure measured at the proximal airways is equal to the end-expiratory alveolar pressure ($PEEP_{TOT}$). AutoPEEP (aka intrinsic PEEP) is the difference between $PEEP_{TOT}$ and set PEEP (Videos 3.3 and 3.4).

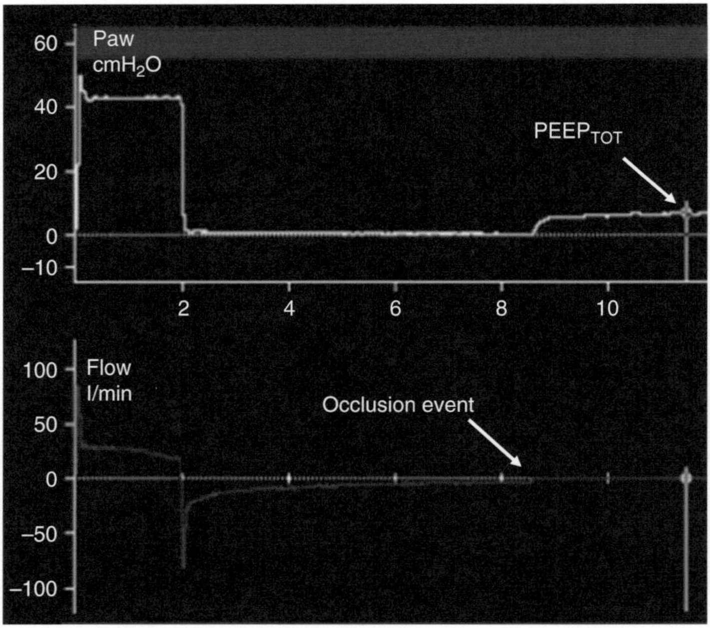

AutoPEEP:

1. Is present if the end-expiratory flow is not zero
2. Can be measured on the pressure curve during an expiratory hold maneuver
3. Is calculated from $PEEP_{TOT}$ and set PEEP
4. Is associated with a long expiratory time constant
5. All of the above

3.14 AutoPEEP Without Dynamic Hyperinflation

AutoPEEP is generally associated with *dynamic hyperinflation*, i.e., a failure to complete full expiration. However, some patients may demonstrate a $PEEP_{TOT}$ higher than set PEEP with complete expiration. In this case, it is due to a load on the chest wall such as severe increased abdominal hypertension (Video 3.5).

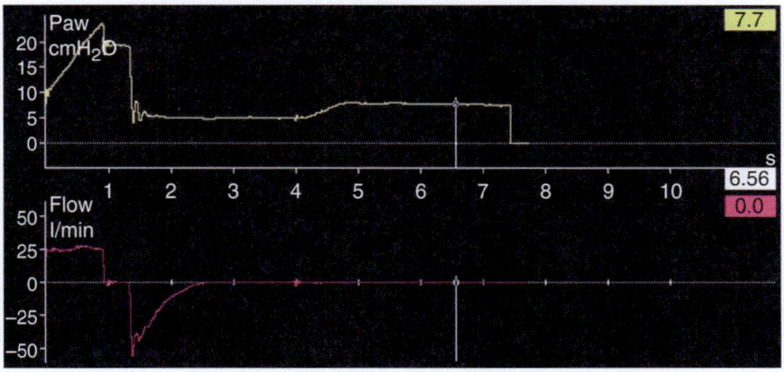

AutoPEEP without dynamic hyperinflation occurs in the case of:

1. Increased intra-abdominal pressure
2. Lung emphysema
3. Acute severe asthma
4. Reverse triggering
5. A large pleural effusion

3.15 Effect of Bronchodilators

Bronchodilators are used to *decrease resistance* in COPD and asthma patients. A positive effect is the result of decreasing airway resistance as demonstrated by an increase in expiratory flow, a shortening of the expiratory time constant, and a decrease in autoPEEP.

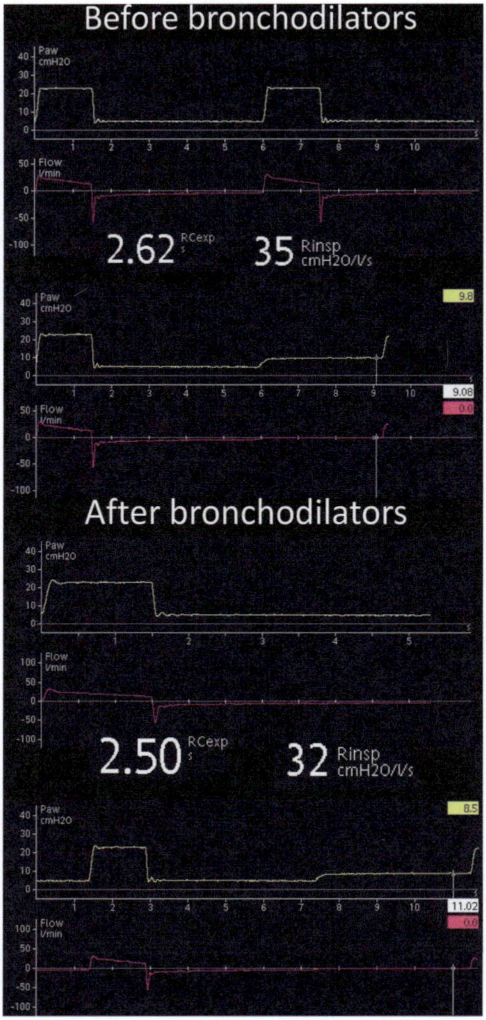

Post-bronchodilator curves in PC show all these figures *except*:

1. Higher peak inspiratory flow
2. Lower plateau pressure
3. Higher peak expiratory flow
4. Shorter time to exhale
5. A shorter expiratory time constant

3.16 Pressure Curve During Expiration

The pressure curve during expiration does not provide information about the patient; instead it mainly *reflects the status of the exhalation valve.* If the exhalation valve demonstrates significant airflow resistance, the pressure drops at the beginning of expiration will be smooth. If the exhalation valve is leaking, the expiratory pressure will be lower than set PEEP.

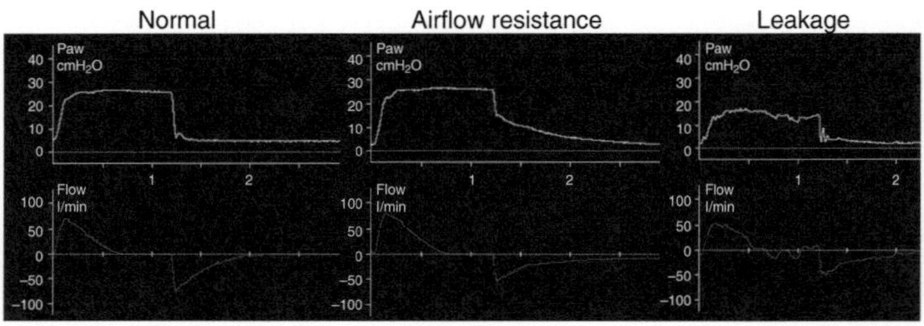

The pressure curve during expiration:

1. Is equal to alveolar pressure
2. Should be equal to set PEEP
3. Is increased in the case of autoPEEP
4. Is increased in the case of exhalation-valve leakage
5. Provide information about the patient's condition

Responses

3.1 2

3.2 5

3.3 2, except if there is intrinsic PEEP

3. End-inspiratory pause decreases a little bit elastic recoil pressure due to viscoelastic relaxation of lung tissues

3.4 4

3.5 1

3.6 3

3.7 1

2. Elastic recoil pressure is decreased in case of COPD patients with lung emphysema. Lung emphysema increases static compliance

5. It depends on RC_{EXP}

3.8 3

3.9 5

3.10 3

3.11 2

3.12 2

3.13 5

3. AutoPEEP is underestimated if set PEEP is increased. However, the mechanism causing autoPEEP is unchanged. Hence, autoPEEP should be measured with low set PEEP

3.14 1

3.15 2

3.16 2

Suggested Readings

Bigatello LM, Davignon KR, et al. Respiratory mechanics and ventilator waveforms in the patient with acute lung injury. Respir Care. 2005;50:235–45.

Blanch L, Bernabé F, et al. Measurement of air trapping, intrinsic positive end-expiratory pressure, and dynamic hyperinflation in mechanically ventilated patients. Respir Care. 2005;50:110–23.

Brochard L. Intrinsic (or auto-) PEEP during controlled mechanical ventilation. Intensive Care Med. 2002a;28:1376–8.

Brochard L. Intrinsic (or auto-) positive end-expiratory pressure during spontaneous or assisted ventilation. Intensive Care Med. 2002b;28:1552–4.

Brunner JX, Laubsher T, et al. Simple method to measure total expiratory time constant based on passive expiratory flow-volume curve. Crit Care Med. 1995;23:1117–22.

Dhand R. Ventilator graphics and respiratory mechanics in the patient with obstructive lung disease. Respir Care. 2005;50:246–61.

Georgopoulos D, Prinianakis G, et al. Bedside waveforms interpretation as a tool to identify patient-ventilator asynchronies. Intensive Care Med. 2006;32:34–47.

Iotti G, Braschi A. Measurement of respiratory mechanics during mechanical ventilation. Rhäzüns, Switzerland: Hamilton Medical Scientific Library; 1999.

Kondili E, Alexopoulou C, et al. Pattern of lung emptying and expiratory resistance in mechanically ventilated patients with chronic obstructive pulmonary disease. Intensive Care Med. 2004;30:1311–8.

Lourens MS, Van Den Berg B, et al. Expiratory time constants in mechanically ventilated patients with and without COPD. Intensive Care Med. 2000;26:1612–8.

Maltais F, Reissmann H, et al. Comparison of static and dynamic measurements of intrinsic PEEP in mechanically ventilated patients. Am J Respir Crit Care Med. 1994;150:1318–24.

Marini JJ. Dynamic hyperinflation and auto-positive end-expiratory pressure: lessons learned over 30 years. Am J Respir Crit Care Med. 2011;184:756–62.

Mauri T, Bellani G, et al. Regional distribution of air trapping in chronic obstructive pulmonary disease. Am J Respir Crit Care Med. 2013;188:1466–7.

Ranieri VM, Grasso S, et al. Auto-positive end-expiratory pressure and dynamic hyperinflation. Clin Chest Med. 1996;17:379–94.

Volta CA, Marangoni E, et al. Respiratory mechanics by least squares fitting in mechanically ventilated patients: application on flow-limited COPD patients. Intensive Care Med. 2002;28:48–52.

Chapter 4
Assisted and Spontaneous Modes

4.1 Pressure Support

4.1.1 Normal Curves

The mode called pressure support is a *particular type of PC in which all breaths are spontaneous* (i.e., patient triggered and patient cycled). The pressure may be shaped by an adjustable pressure rise time setting. The subsequent inspiratory flow depends on the inspiratory time constant and the patient's inspiratory effort. Inspiration stops when the set cycle threshold is reached (expiratory trigger sensitivity). The cycle threshold is set as a percentage of the peak inspiratory flow. The point at which the cycle threshold is reached depends on the inspiratory time constant; hence cycling is a patient-initiated event, even if inspiration is entirely passive after triggering (Video 4.1).

Electronic Supplementary Material The online version of this chapter (https://doi.org/10.1007/978-3-319-58655-7_4) contains supplementary material, which is available to authorized users.

J.-M. Arnal, *Monitoring Mechanical Ventilation Using Ventilator Waveforms*, https://doi.org/10.1007/978-3-319-58655-7_4

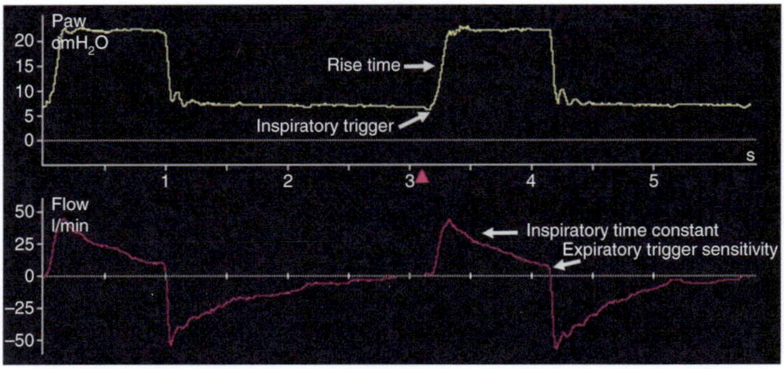

All of the statements regarding pressure support are true *except*:

1. The inspiratory trigger event is visible on the pressure curve
2. The inspiratory flow is variable depending on patient inspiratory effort
3. The inspiratory time is preset
4. The expiratory cycle threshold is based on flow
5. The respiratory rate is controlled by the patient

4.1.2 Inspiratory Trigger

The *patient's inspiratory effort* is detected as a deformation of the pressure or flow waveform. Pressure triggering requires patient effort to decrease the airway pressure from PEEP down to a preset threshold. During the pre-trigger phase, airway pressure decreases and flow is zero. With flow triggering, a continuous bias flow is maintained through the ventilator circuit. When the patient generates an inspiratory effort, a fraction of the base flow deviates to the patient. The drop in expiratory flow below the base flow is the signal for triggering inspiration. During the pre-trigger phase, airway pressure decreases and flow increases slightly.

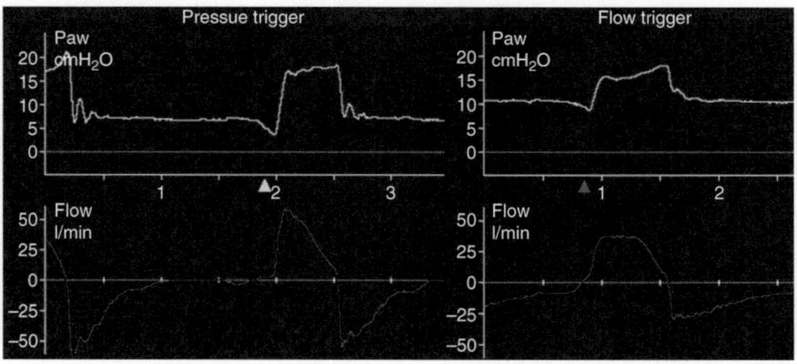

Inspiratory trigger:

1. Is indicated by an increase in pressure before the mechanical breath
2. Is not visible on the pressure curve if a flow trigger is used
3. Always increases flow at initiation of patient's effort
4. Demonstrates different flow curve during the pre-trigger phase depending on the trigger mechanism
5. Is equivalent with a flow or a pressure trigger mechanism

4.1.3 Trigger Effort

The patient's effort to trigger a breath is indicated by the *depth of the pressure deflection* below the baseline, and the time during which the pressure remains below the baseline. The depth of the pressure deflection can be more negative than the set trigger pressure if the patient has a strong respiratory drive.

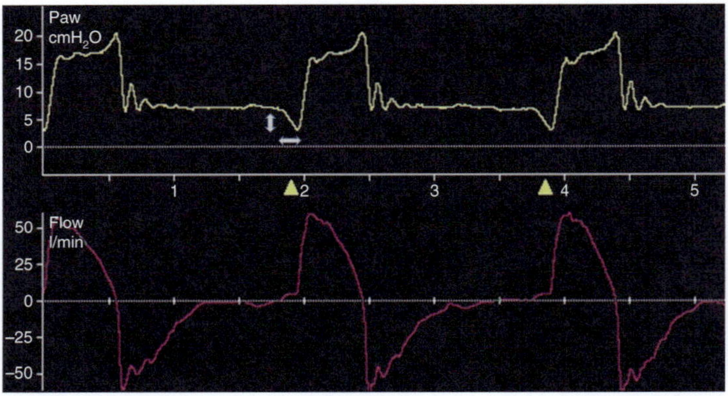

A deep deflection in pressure during the triggering phase indicates all these *except*:

1. An inadequate trigger sensitivity setting
2. The need to increase pressure support
3. Patient-ventilator asynchrony
4. The need to use a flow-triggering system
5. A high respiratory drive

4.1.4 Inspiratory Trigger Time

Inspiratory trigger time is the time that elapses *between the initial patient effort and the start of inspiratory flow* from the ventilator. The patient's effort starts when the airway pressure decreases below PEEP and/or the expiratory flow deviates suddenly from its trajectory (e.g., in the presence of gas trapping). This abrupt deviation of flow from its trajectory may also indicate relaxation of the expiratory muscles if expiration is active. Mechanical assistance starts when airway pressure rises above PEEP.

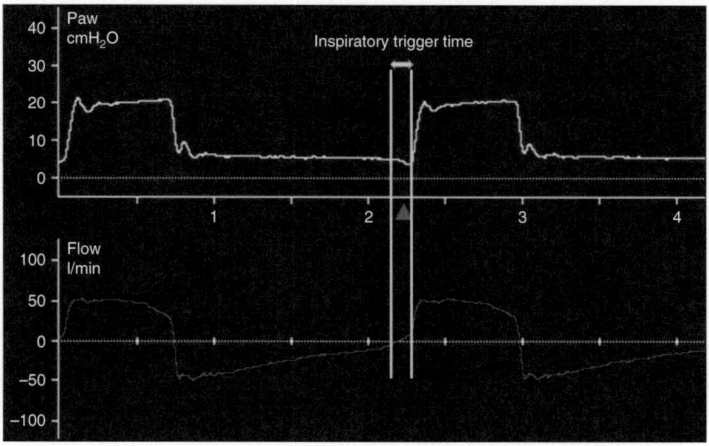

Initiation of the patient's inspiratory effort is determined by:

1. An increase in flow above the baseline
2. An increase in pressure
3. A decrease in pressure below zero
4. A deviation of flow from its trajectory
5. The triangle below the pressure curve

4.1.5 Inspiratory Delay Time

Inspiratory delay time is the time that elapses *between the initial patient effort and the pressure returning to baseline*. It is the sum of the inspiratory trigger time and the time needed to return pressure to baseline (post-triggering phase), which depends on inspiratory pressure setting, pressure rise time, and ventilator pneumatics.

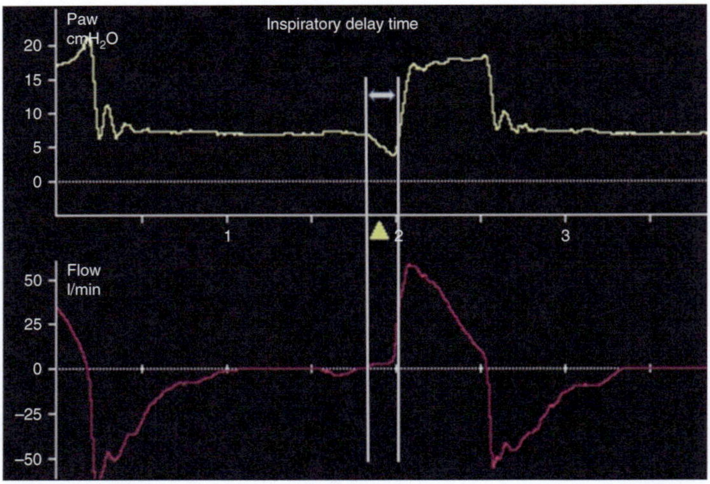

Inspiratory delay time depends on all variables *except*:

1. The inspiratory trigger sensitivity setting
2. The expiratory trigger sensitivity setting
3. The presence of autoPEEP
4. The pressure rise time setting
5. Ventilator pneumatics

4.1.6 *Ineffective Inspiratory Efforts*

Ineffective inspiratory efforts appear on the flow curve as a *sudden deviation of the expiratory flow* toward the baseline (upward convexity) and a concomitant drop in airway pressure toward the baseline (upward concavity). Ineffective inspiratory efforts occur in the case of low respiratory drive and/or dynamic hyperinflation (perhaps due to excessive inspiratory pressure) (Video 4.2).

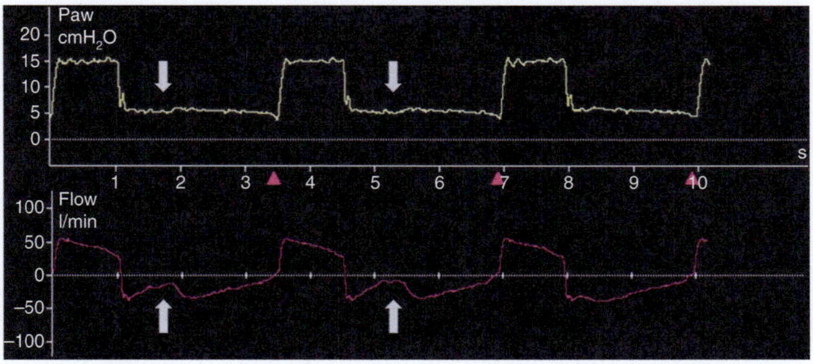

All statements regarding ineffective inspiratory efforts are true *except*:

1. Occur during expiration
2. Decrease airway pressure
3. Direct the flow toward the baseline
4. Are commonly associated with dynamic hyperinflation
5. Can be detected only through esophageal pressure measurement

4.1.7 Cardiac Oscillations

Flow distortion due to cardiac oscillations may be confused with ineffective inspiratory efforts. The short duration (less than 0.3 s) and the *rapid frequency* of these distortions equal to the heart rate suggest cardiac oscillations rather than ineffective inspiratory efforts.

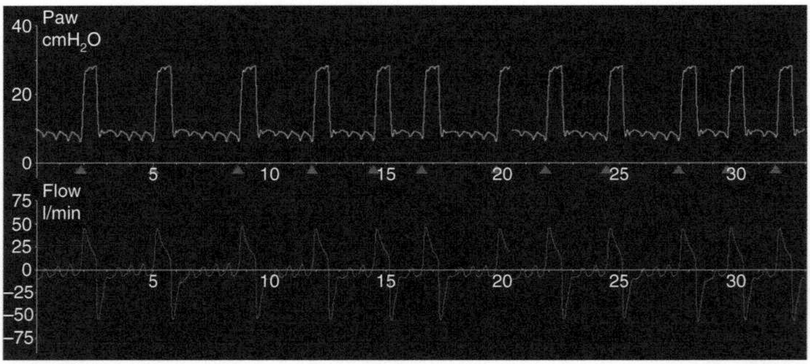

Cardiac oscillations can be distinguished from ineffective inspiratory efforts because they:

1. Occur several times during expiratory time
2. Are smaller in size
3. Have a frequency that is close to the heart rate
4. Are able to trigger a mechanical breath
5. All the above

4.1.8 Autotriggering

Autotriggering during pressure support occurs when *inspiration is triggered inadvertently*, without the patient's inspiratory effort. Autotriggering is associated with a low respiratory drive and respiratory rate and the absence of dynamic hyperinflation. It can be caused by circuit leaks, the presence of water in the ventilator circuit, and cardiac oscillations. The absence of an initial pressure drop during the pre-trigger phase may be indicative of autotriggering. Triggering that occurs synchronously with cardiac oscillations suggests autotriggering. The inspiratory flow curve of an autotriggered breath differs substantially from that of patient-triggered breaths because the patient doesn't make an active inspiratory effort—the peak inspiratory flow is lower and the inspiratory time is shorter (Video 4.3).

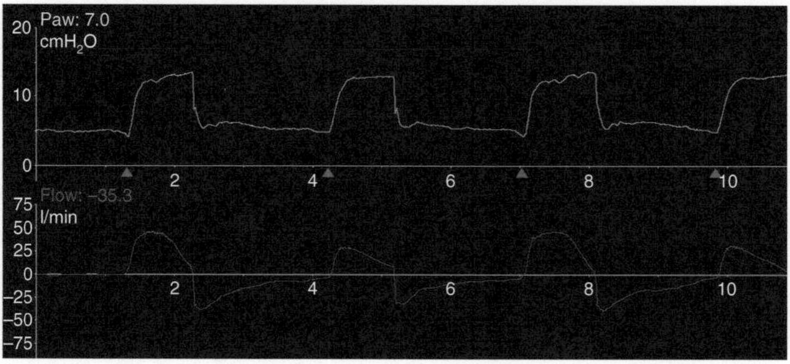

Autotriggering can be caused by all these *except*:

1. Cardiac oscillations
2. Water in the ventilator circuit
3. Dynamic hyperinflation
4. Too sensitive setting for the inspiratory trigger
5. Bronchopleural fistula

4.1.9 Double Triggering

Double (or multiple) triggering is defined as *two (or more) assisted breaths without expiration* between them. Double triggering can be easily identified on both the pressure and flow curves. It is caused either by premature cycling of the first breath or by insufficient pressure support. The patient is still making an inspiratory effort when the first inspiration stops and the second inspiration is triggered, hence the lack of an expiration between the two inspirations. Double triggering is associated with a fast pressure rise time, premature cycling, and a high respiratory drive (Video 4.4).

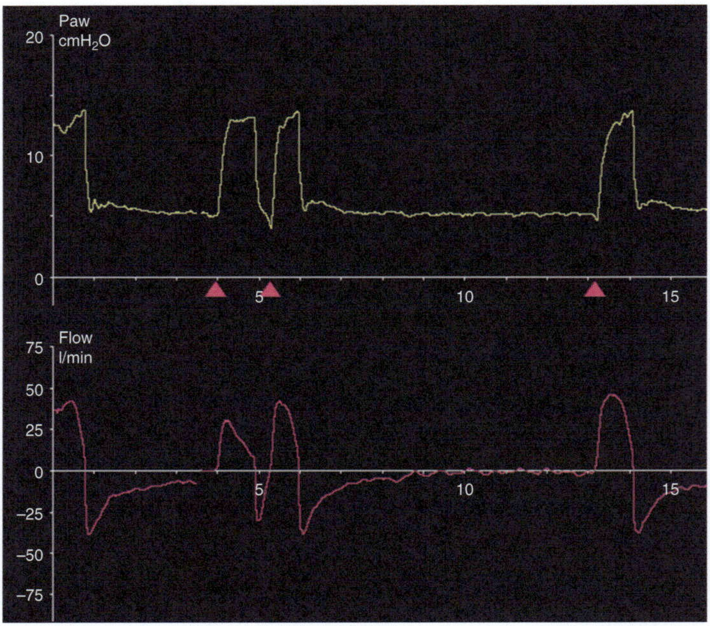

Double triggering can be avoided by:

1. Decreasing pressure support
2. Prolonging the mechanical breath
3. Lowering the setting for inspiratory trigger sensitivity
4. Increasing the rise time
5. Increasing PEEP

4.1.10 *Pressure Rise Time*

Pressure rise time is the *time to increase pressure from* PEEP *to* P_{INSP} at the onset of inspiration. Pressure rise time is adjustable for most PC modes, so the delivery of breaths can be adjusted to meet the patient's demand and clinical condition. The shorter the rise time, the higher the peak inspiratory flow. As the expiratory trigger sensitivity is a fixed percentage of the peak inspiratory flow, pressure rise time setting also influences insufflation time, i.e., the duration of the mechanical breath.

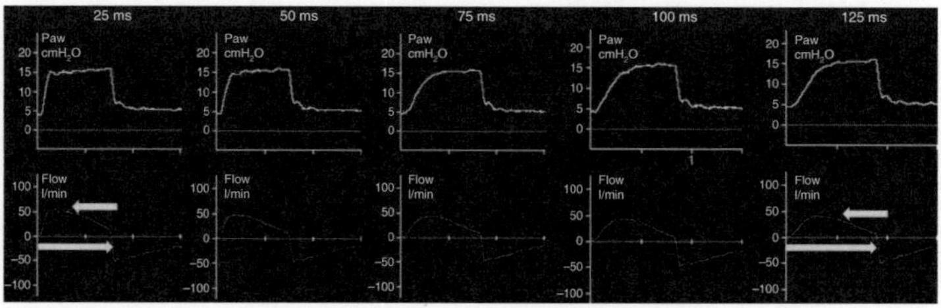

All statements regarding pressure rise time are true *except*:

1. Is the pressurization rate at the initiation of the inspiratory phase
2. Should be as fast as possible
3. Influences the peak inspiratory flow
4. Influences the work of breathing
5. Should be set according to respiratory mechanics and respiratory drive

4.1.11 Peak Inspiratory Flow

In pressure support mode, the peak inspiratory flow results from interaction between set inspiratory pressure, pressure rise time, patient effort and compliance, and resistance of the respiratory system. The peak inspiratory flow *should match the patient's needs* in order to be comfortable and decrease work of breathing.

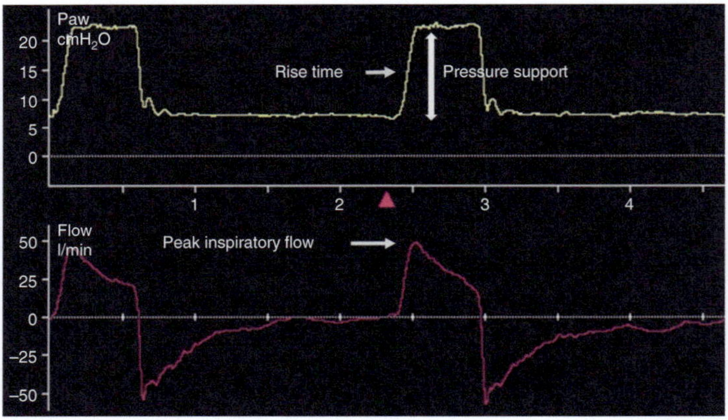

The peak inspiratory flow depends on all variables *except*:

1. PEEP
2. Inspiratory pressure setting
3. The patient's inspiratory effort
4. The rise time setting
5. Respiratory mechanics

4.1.12 *Pressure Overshoot*

If the pressure rise time is set very short and respiratory-system impedance is relatively high, the airway pressure at the onset of inspiration may *exceed the target* and create a pressure overshoot. If this overshoot is large enough, it may be associated with a flow overshoot at the same time, which exposes the patient to premature cycling. In addition, a flow overshoot may activate a flow-related inspiratory terminating reflex that shortens neural inspiration and induces brief, shallow inspiratory efforts. A slower pressure rise time may reduce or eliminate the overshoot.

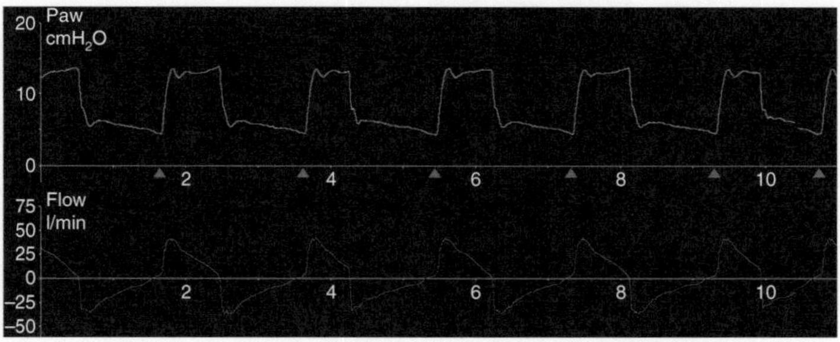

All statements regarding overshoot at the onset of inspiration are true *except*:

1. Appears on the pressure curve
2. May appear on the flow curve
3. Is due to a high respiratory drive
4. Is associated with a fast pressure rise time
5. Is associated with low compliance

4.1.13 Flow Overshoot

If a flow overshoot occurs at the onset of inspiration without a pressure overshoot, it means that the *patient's inspiratory effort has stopped suddenly*. This occurs when there is a long inspiratory trigger delay. The patient's inspiratory effort starts long before the mechanical breath is delivered and stops soon after the beginning of mechanical breath.

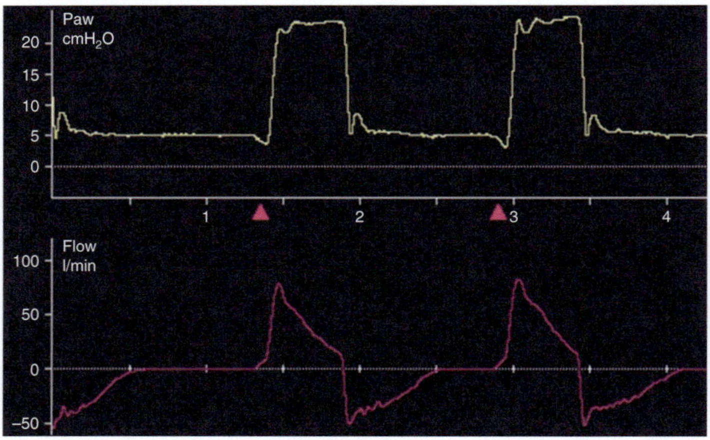

A flow overshoot at the onset of inspiration without a pressure overshoot is associated with:

1. High resistance
2. A high respiratory drive
3. Low compliance
4. Dynamic hyperinflation
5. A long inspiratory delay

4.1.14 Shape of Inspiratory Flow

After the initial peak inspiratory flow, inspiratory flow declines according to an exponential curve if there is no active inspiratory effort. Kinetic of the inspiratory flow decline depends on the *inspiratory time constant*, i.e., the respiratory mechanics. If compliance is low, the flow declines rapidly and the insufflation time is short. Conversely, if the resistance increases, the flow declines slowly and the insufflation time is prolonged.

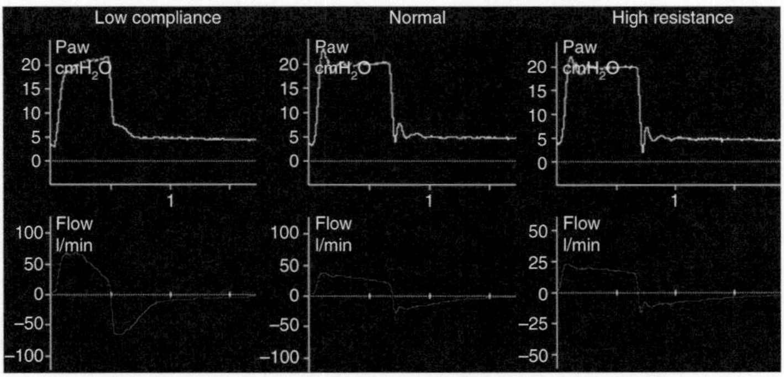

The shape of the inspiratory flow in pressure support depends on all these variables *except*:

1. Resistance
2. Inspiratory pressure setting
3. Compliance
4. Dynamic hyperinflation
5. Patient effort

4.1.15 Inspiratory Effort

Any *deviation of inspiratory flow* from the exponential declining pattern indicates a respiratory muscle effort (inspiratory or expiratory). Rounded or constant inspiratory flow suggests a significant inspiratory effort during insufflation and indicates insufficient pressure support. Conversely, a change in the slope of inspiratory flow toward the baseline suggests an expiratory muscle contraction during insufflation (or just relaxation of a large effort), which is caused by excessive pressure support or prolonged mechanical insufflation.

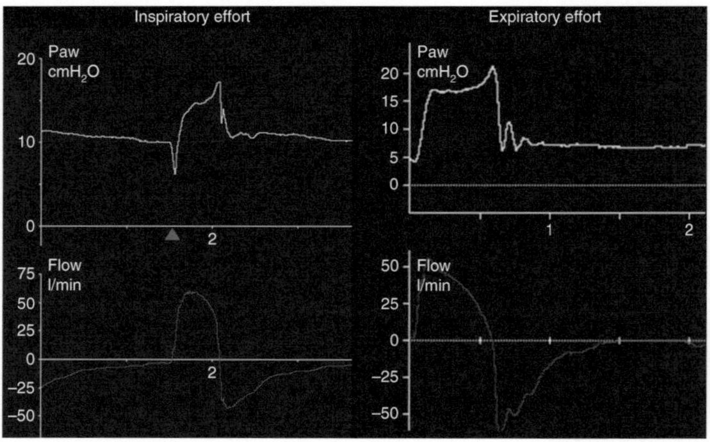

Inspiratory effort during insufflation is indicated by:

1. A rounded shape of the inspiratory flow
2. An exponential decline in flow
3. A change in the flow slope toward the baseline
4. A constant flow during insufflation
5. A pressure overshot at the onset of inspiration

4.1.16 Expiratory Trigger Sensitivity

The cycle threshold during pressure support is set using what is sometimes called the expiratory trigger sensitivity (ETS). The setting is calibrated as a *fixed percentage of the peak inspiratory flow*. A high threshold (high percentage) results in a short insufflation time. Conversely, a low threshold results in a long insufflation time. However, as the peak inspiratory flow may change from breath to breath depending on the patient's inspiratory effort, the inspiratory time changes randomly from breath to breath. The clinician should adjust the expiratory trigger sensitivity to match the apparent average "neural inspiratory time" to optimize patient-ventilator synchrony (Video 4.5).

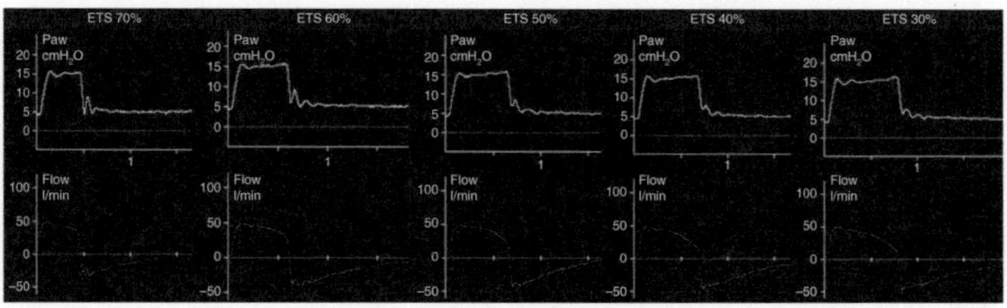

Inspiratory time in pressure support depends on all these variables *except*:

1. The preset I:E ratio
2. The patient's inspiratory effort
3. The inspiratory pressure setting
4. Respiratory mechanics
5. The expiratory trigger sensitivity setting

4.1.17 Optimal Expiratory Trigger Sensitivity Setting

The optimal expiratory trigger sensitivity *depends on respiratory mechanics*. In patients with increased resistance and a long inspiratory time constant, a high percentage of expiratory trigger sensitivity is preferred in order to provide a conventional insufflation time. Conversely, in patients with low compliance and a short inspiratory time constant, a low percentage of expiratory trigger sensitivity is preferred in order to allow enough time for insufflation.

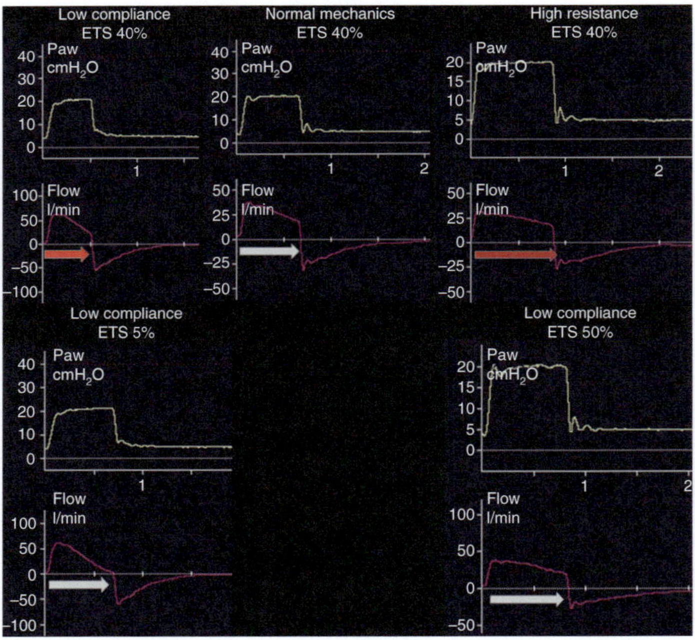

The following are optimal expiratory trigger sensitivity; all are true *except*:

1. 25–40% for a normal-lung condition
2. Above 40% in the case of obstructive disease
3. 50% in the case of low compliance
4. 25–40% in the case of a mixed condition (increased resistance and decreased compliance)
5. Below 25% in the case of restrictive disease

4.1.18 *Early Cycling*

Early cycling occurs when flow from the ventilator ends while the *patient is still making an inspiratory effort*. Early cycling distorts both the flow and pressure waveforms at the onset of expiration. The flow curve demonstrates a smaller peak expiratory flow, followed by an abrupt initial reversal in the expiratory flow. The expiratory flow slope has a rapid deflection toward zero, indicating that the patient's inspiratory effort is prolonged. The pressure decreases rapidly from inspiratory pressure to a value below PEEP, with an upward convexity indicating the patient's inspiratory effort. In an exaggerated condition, continuation of the patient's inspiratory effort may result in double triggering.

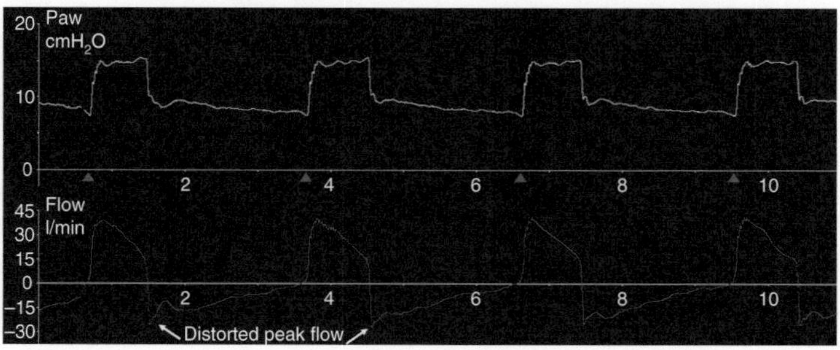

Early cycling:

1. Decreases the respiratory rate
2. Increases tidal volume
3. Decreases work of breathing
4. Decreases insufflation time
5. Induces active expiratory effort

4.1.19 Delayed Cycling

Delayed cycling occurs when the assisted breath is *prolonged beyond the end of the patient's inspiratory effort.* Delayed cycling is indicated by distortions in both the flow and pressure waveforms at the end of insufflation. The flow curve demonstrates a change in the slope toward the baseline, indicating either an abrupt relaxation of the inspiratory muscle or a contraction of the expiratory muscle. Simultaneously, the pressure curve rises above the target at the end of insufflation.

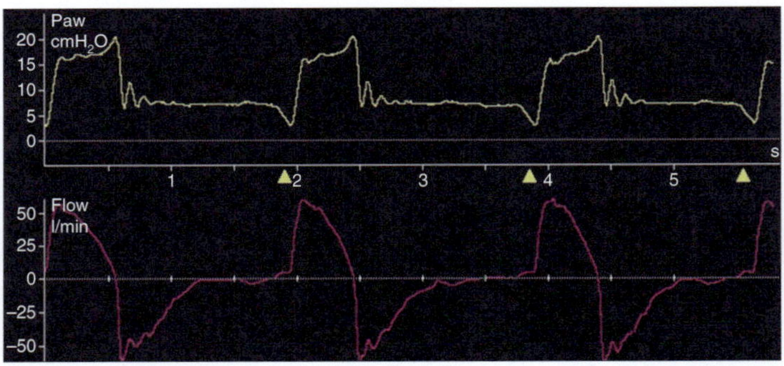

Delayed cycling:

1. Decreases tidal volume
2. Decreases insufflation time
3. May reduce dynamic hyperinflation
4. Occurs mainly in a low-compliance system
5. Is signaled by a pressure rise at the end of insufflation

4.1.20 *Delayed Cycling and Strong Inspiratory Effort*

Delayed cycling and relaxation of a strong inspiratory effort both induce a *rise in pressure at the end of insufflation*. The cause can be ascertained by observing the inspiratory flow curve. If the inspiratory flow curve has a rounded shape or shows a constant flow, rise in pressure is probably due to an abrupt relaxation of the inspiratory muscles. In this case, increasing the pressure support may be efficient. If the inspiratory flow curve demonstrates a change from the usual fast exponential decline to a slow exponential decline, this indicates the end of the inspiratory effort and the beginning of a secondary phase of passive inflation. Conversely, a change in the slope of the inspiratory flow curve toward baseline indicates activation of the expiratory muscles. In these last two cases, reducing the insufflation time by setting a higher level of expiratory trigger sensitivity may improve patient-ventilator synchrony.

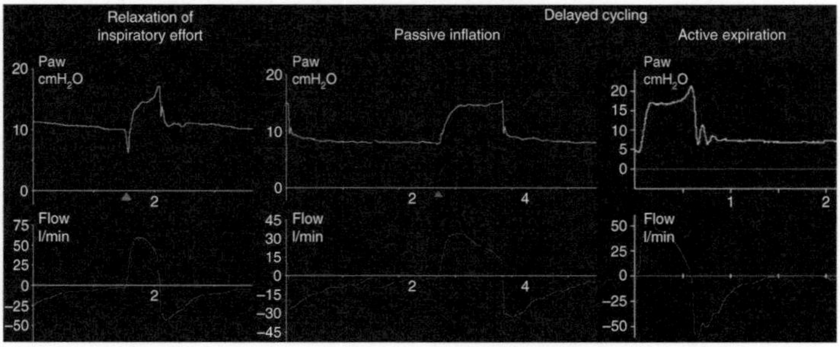

Rise in pressure at the end of insufflation is due to:

1. Inspiratory effort longer than inspiratory flow
2. Expiratory trigger sensitivity too high
3. An inadequate PEEP setting
4. A prolonged inspiratory trigger delay
5. Relaxation of a large inspiratory effort

4.2 Volume Assist Control

4.2.1 Normal Pressure Curve

In VAC modes, the pressure curve is *linear* for passive inflation or for inspiratory effort only large enough to trigger inspiration (indicated by drop in pressure just before the start of flow) (Video 4.6).

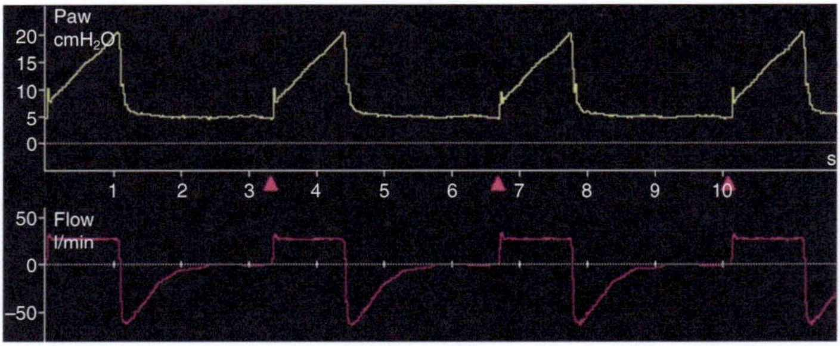

In VAC, which statement is not true about airway pressure?

1. Airway pressure decreases in the pre-trigger phase
2. Pressure increases rapidly at the onset of insufflation depending on the airway resistance
3. The inspiratory time depends on the patient's effort
4. Peak pressure depends on PEEP, tidal volume, compliance, and resistance
5. The respiratory rate is controlled by the patient

4.2.2 Flow Starvation

In VAC mode, the inspiratory flow is controlled by the ventilator. The pressure curve can be used to assess *whether the flow is adequate*. Any patient inspiratory effort will distort the pressure curve during its ascending part (upward concavity). The decrease in mean inspiratory pressure indicates that the ventilator is doing less work on the patient (i.e., providing less support for the work of breathing). In the worst case, if flow from the ventilator is less than what the patient would get if not connected to the ventilator, then airway pressure drops below the baseline, and the patient is actually doing work on the ventilator. This situation has been called "flow starvation."

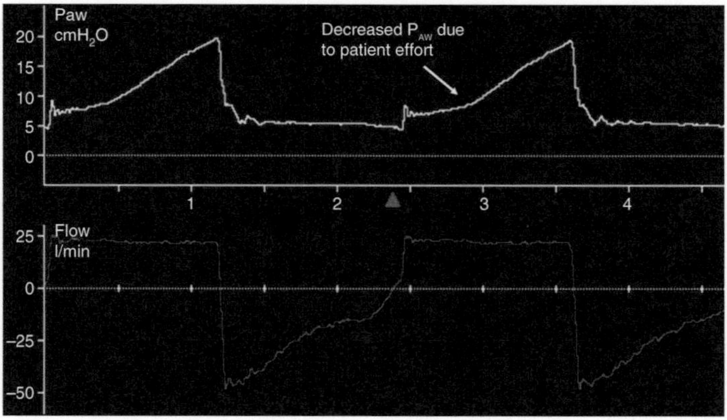

In VAC mode:

1. Flow starvation is associated with a higher tidal volume
2. The larger the inspiratory effort, the higher the mean inspiratory pressure
3. The lower the mean inspiratory pressure, the less assistance from the ventilator
4. Flow starvation is demonstrated by a distortion of the flow curve
5. Flow starvation is indicated when pressure falls below PEEP

Responses

4.1.1 3

4.1.2 4

4.1.3 2

4.1.4 4

4.1.5 2

4.1.6 5

4.1.7 5

4.1.8 3

4.1.9 2

4.1.10 2

4. Slow pressure rise times are associated with increased work of breathing

4.1.11 1

4.1.12 3

4.1.13 5

4.1.14 4

4.1.15 1

4.1.16 1

4.1.17 3

4.1.18 4

4.1.19 5

4.1.20 5

4.2.1 3

4.2.2 5

Suggested Readings

Aslanian P, El Atrous S, et al. Effects of flow triggering on breathing effort during partial ventilatory support. Am J Respir Crit Care Med. 1998;157:135–43.

Chiumello D, Pelosi P, et al. Effect of different inspiratory rise time and cycling off criteria during pressure support ventilation in patients recovering from acute lung injury. Crit Care Med. 2003;31:2604–10.

Dhand R. Ventilator graphics and respiratory mechanics in the patient with obstructive lung disease. Respir Care. 2005;50:246–61.

Du HL, Yamada Y. Expiratory asynchrony. Respir Care Clin N Am. 2005;11:265–80.

Fernandez R, Mendez M et al (1999) Effect of ventilator flow rate on respiratory timing in normal humans. Am J Respir Crit Care Med 159:710–9.

Georgopoulos D, Prinianakis G, et al. Bedside waveforms interpretation as a tool to identify patient-ventilator asynchronies. Intensive Care Med. 2006;32:34–47.

Grinnan DC, Truwit JD. Clinical review: respiratory mechanics in spontaneous and assisted ventilation. Crit Care. 2005;9:472–84.

Hess DR. Ventilator waveforms and the physiology of pressure support ventilation. Respir Care. 2005;50:166–86.

Hoff FC, Tucci MR, et al. Cycling-off modes during pressure support ventilation: effects on breathing pattern, patient effort, and comfort. J Crit Care. 2014;29:380–5.

Kondili E, Prinianakis G, et al. Patient-ventilator interaction. Br J Anaesth. 2003;91:106–19.

Mojoli F, Iotti GA, et al. Is the ventilator switching from inspiration to expiration at the right time? Look at waveforms! Intensive Care Med. 2016;42:914–5.

Nilsestuen JO, Hargett KD. Using ventilator graphics to identify patient-ventilator asynchrony. Respir Care. 2005;50:202–34.

Parthasarathy S, Jubran A, et al. Cycling of inspiratory and expiratory muscle groups with the ventilator in airflow limitation. Am J Respir Crit Care Med. 1998;158:1471–8.

Prinianakis G, Kondili E, et al. Effects of the flow waveform method of triggering and cycling on patient-ventilator interaction during pressure support. Intensive Care Med. 2003;29:1950–9.

Prinianakis G, Plataki M, et al. Effects of relaxation of inspiratory muscles on ventilator pressure during pressure support. Intensive Care Med. 2008;34:70–4.

Racca F, Squadrone V, et al. Patient-ventilator interaction during the triggering phase. Respir Care Clin N Am. 2005;11:225–45.

Tassaux D, Gainnier M, et al. Impact of expiratory trigger setting on delayed cycling and inspiratory muscle workload. Am J Respir Crit Care Med. 2005;172:1283–9.

Thille AW, Rodriguez P, et al. Patient-ventilator asynchrony during assisted mechanical ventilation. Intensive Care Med. 2006;32:1515–22.

Thille AW, Cabello B, et al. Reduction of patient-ventilator asynchrony by reducing tidal volume during pressure-support ventilation. Intensive Care Med. 2008;34:1477–86.

Tobin MJ, Jubran A, et al. Patient-ventilator interaction. Am J Respir Crit Care Med. 2001;163:1059–63.

Tusman G, Suarez-Sipmann F, et al. Pulmonary blood flow generates cardiogenic oscillations. Respir Physiol Neurobiol. 2009;167:247–54.

Yamada Y, Du HL. Analysis of the mechanisms of expiratory asynchrony in pressure support ventilation: a mathematical approach. J Appl Physiol. 2000;88:2143–50.

Chapter 5
Noninvasive Ventilation

5.1 NIV in Pressure Support Mode

Noninvasive ventilation (NIV) is frequently applied using the pressure support mode. The *curves are characteristic of PC modes* in general, i.e., relatively constant inspiratory pressure with decreasing flow waveform (for passive inspiration). Particular to NIV are the unintentional leaks and upper airway obstructions that can be detected on the curves. The curves also show patient-ventilator asynchronies, which are common in NIV (Video 5.1)

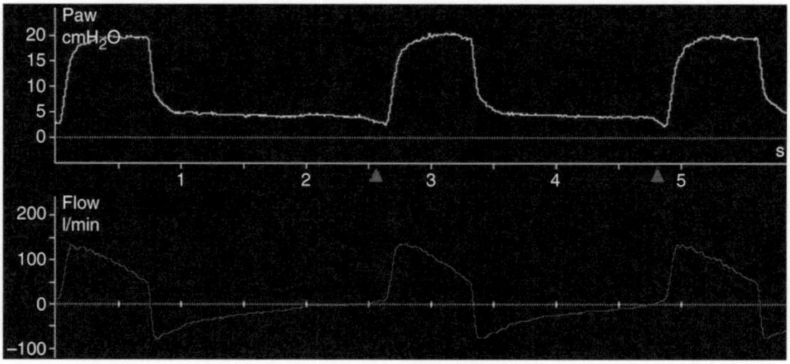

Electronic Supplementary Material The online version of this chapter (https://doi.org/10.1007/978-3-319-58655-7_5) contains supplementary material, which is available to authorized users.

J.-M. Arnal, *Monitoring Mechanical Ventilation Using Ventilator Waveforms*, https://doi.org/10.1007/978-3-319-58655-7_5

All these statements regarding curves in NIV using the PS mode are true *except*:

1. Curves are similar to those seen in intubated patients ventilated in PC mode
2. Curves can show unintentional leaks
3. Curves can't be interpreted because of the leaks
4. Curves may show upper airway obstruction
5. Curves may demonstrate patient-ventilator asynchrony

5.2 Unintentional Leaks

An *increase in inspiratory flow* and a *decrease in expiratory flow* may point to the presence of unintentional leaks. This can be confirmed by making a visual comparison of the area below the curves of the inspiratory and expiratory flow, respectively. If there are no unintentional leaks, the area below the two curves will be similar. However, if the area below the inspiratory flow curve is larger than the area below the expiratory flow curve, it means that part of the inspiratory volume is leakage.

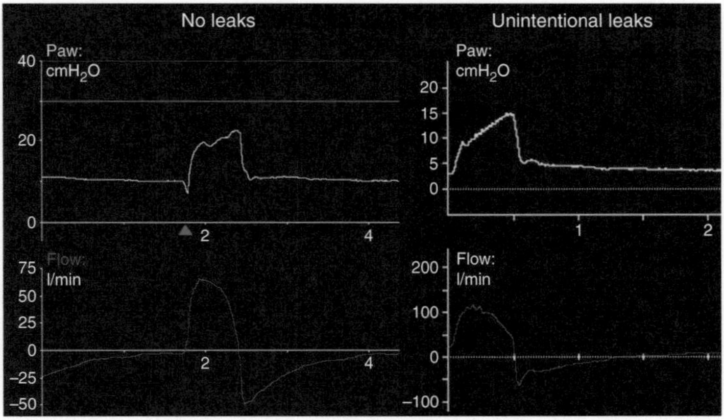

Unintentional leaks are demonstrated:

1. By a high inspiratory flow
2. By a low expiratory flow
3. By a discrepancy between the area below the curve of the inspiratory and expiratory flows respectively
4. By oscillations in the flow curve
5. By a decrease in pressure during insufflation

5.3 Leak Rate

When an inspiratory flow trigger is used, a continuous air leak can be suspected if the *flow is above baseline at the end of expiration*. The leak flow rate can then be measured for a given setting of PEEP. For a continuous leak, the leak flow rate increases when pressure is increased. If the flow curves demonstrate unintentional leaks (discrepancy between the area below the curve of the inspiratory and expiratory flows, respectively) with an end-expiratory flow at the baseline, it means that leaks are not continuous and occur mainly during insufflation, when pressure in the mask increases above a certain leak pressure.

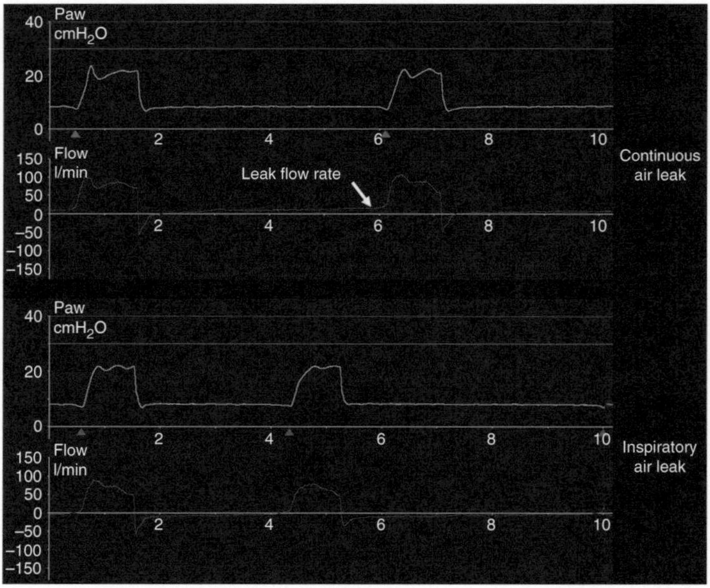

The presence and type of leakage can be determined as follows:

1. A positive flow at the end of expiration suggests continuous leaks
2. A negative flow at the end of expiration occurs if there are no unintentional leaks
3. The flow curve at baseline at the end of expiration indicates continuous leaks
4. The flow curve at baseline at the end of expiration indicates discontinuous leaks
5. An expiratory pressure below PEEP occurs in the case of unintentional leaks from the NIV mask

5.4 Inspiratory Trigger Delay

A drop in end-expiratory pressure signals indicates when patient's inspiratory effort starts. The flow increases at the same time only if a flow-trigger system is used. Pressure and flow abruptly increase when flow delivery starts. Inspiratory trigger delay occurs if the time between the start of the patient's inspiratory effort and the start of inspiratory flow from the ventilator insufflation *is longer than 200 ms*. Inspiratory trigger delay occurs in case of low respiratory drive, dynamic hyperinflation, and/or unintentional leaks.

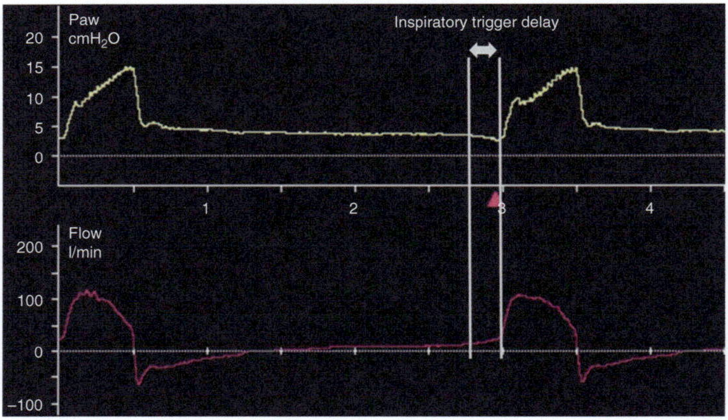

Inspiratory trigger delay is caused by all these *except*:

1. Dynamic hyperinflation
2. Using an inspiratory trigger setting that is not sensitive enough
3. A slow rise time
4. A low respiratory drive
5. Unintentional leaks

5.5 Autotriggering

Autotriggering occurs frequently in NIV in the case of unintentional leaks, when the leak flow rate is higher than the trigger threshold. This is demonstrated by the *absence of any patient effort* at the beginning of insufflation. Autotriggered breaths are shorter, and the peak inspiratory flow is lower in comparison to a patient-triggered breath. Sometimes several autotriggered breaths occur consecutively without full expiration between them that are called multiple triggering (Video 5.2).

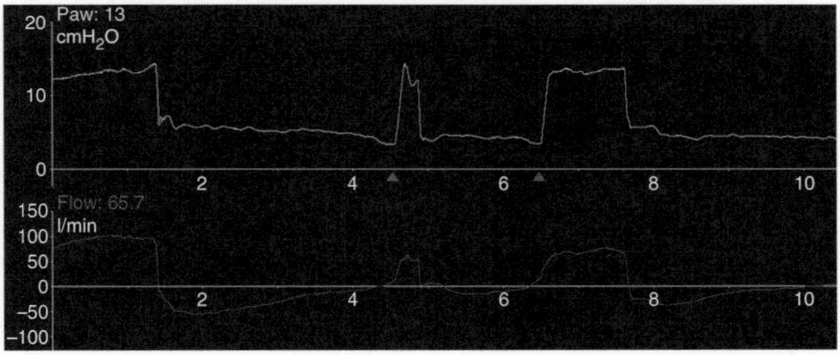

Autotriggering and multiple triggering are indicated by all these *except*:

1. Several breaths triggered rapidly without full expiration between them
2. A high respiratory rate
3. A large drop in pressure before the breath
4. The absence of patient effort at the beginning of the breath
5. A short breath

5.6 Double Triggering

Double triggering consists of *two patient-triggered breaths without expiration* between them and can be seen on the pressure and flow curves. Double triggering occurs in the case of a strong patient inspiratory effort combined with premature cycling.

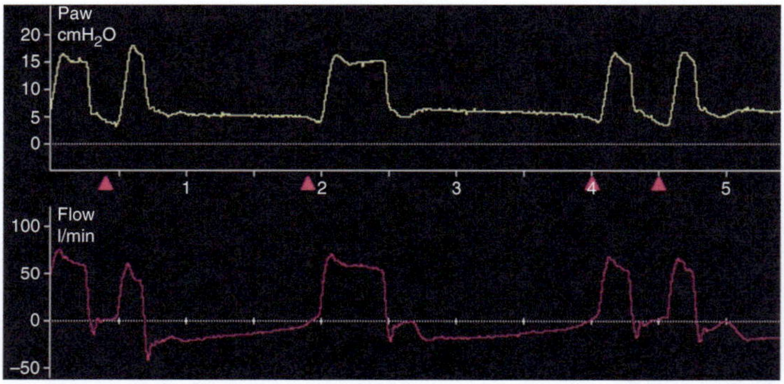

Double triggering is:

1. A ventilator-triggered breath followed by a patient-triggered breath
2. A patient-triggered breath followed by an autotriggered breath
3. A ventilator-triggered followed by an autotriggered breath
4. Two patient-triggered breaths without expiration between them
5. Associated with delayed cycling

5.7 Ineffective Inspiratory Effort

Ineffective inspiratory efforts are common during NIV, especially in the case of unintentional leaks. The *expiratory flow shows a sudden deviation toward the baseline* (upward convexity), and the expiratory pressure simultaneously deviates toward the baseline (upward concavity) (Video 5.3).

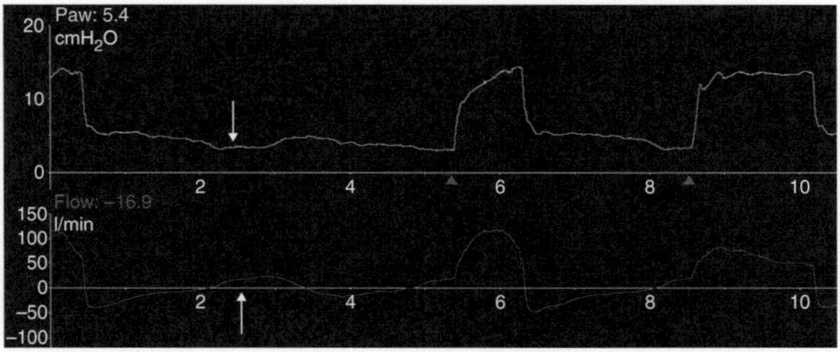

All these statements regarding ineffective inspiratory efforts are true *except*:

1. Occur mainly at the beginning of expiration
2. Occur mainly during the second half of expiration
3. May be hidden by cardiogenic oscillations
4. Are more frequent in the case of unintentional leaks
5. Are displayed on the pressure and flow curves

5.8 Flow Overshoot

Flow overshoot is demonstrated by a *peak of pressure and flow at the beginning of insufflation.* Flow overshoot is caused by high pressure support and a fast pressure rise time and occurs mainly in restrictive disease (low compliance and normal resistance). Flow overshoot is usually quite uncomfortable for the patient. In addition, it may cause premature cycling because the peak inspiratory flow is increased. Furthermore, a high inspiratory flow may activate a reflex that causes a shortening of neural inspiration and results in a short and shallow inspiratory effort or an expiratory effort.

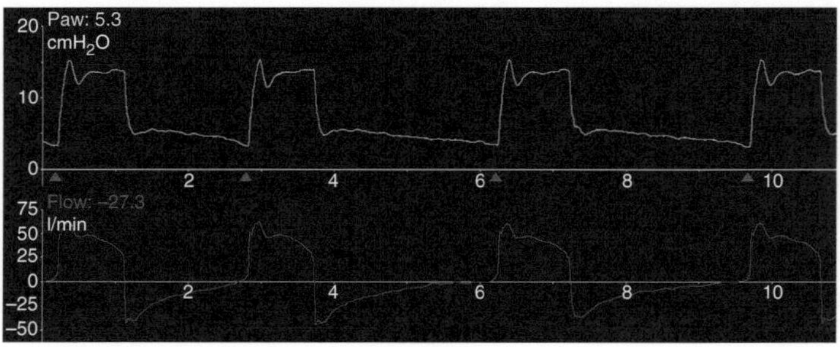

Flow overshoot:

1. Is a peak of pressure at the end of insufflation
2. Is caused by a fast pressure rise time
3. Is caused by unintentional leaks
4. Is a peak of flow at the beginning of expiration
5. Occurs mainly in obstructive patients

5.9 Patient Effort

The inspiratory flow normally has a *triangular shape* with an exponential decline in flow during insufflation for a patient making minimal inspiratory effort. If the patient maintains an inspiratory effort throughout insufflation, the inspiratory flow will have a rounded shape. This means that pressure support may be increased in order to reduce the work of breathing.

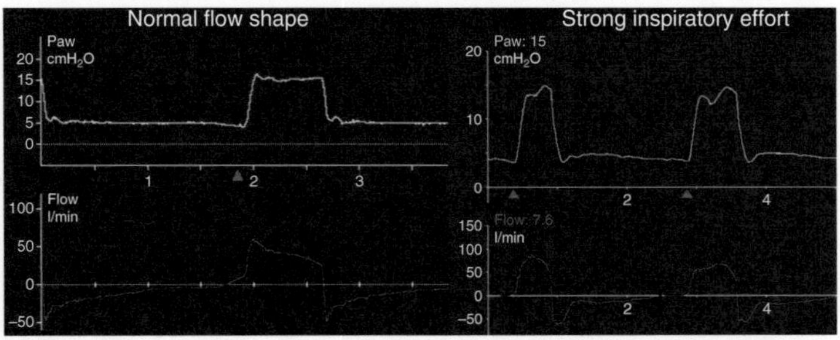

All statements regarding the flow curve during inspiration are true *except*:

1. Flow curve displays an initial peak followed by an exponential decline
2. Flow curve may have a square shape
3. Flow curve has a rounded shape when the patient maintains an inspiratory effort throughout insufflation
4. Flow curve informs indirectly about the work of breathing
5. Flow curve is affected by unintentional leaks

5.10 Leaks and Cycling

The inspiratory flow shape is distorted by unintentional leaks with a *more gradual decline in flow*. Sometimes the leak flow rate may be higher than the set cycle threshold (i.e., a percentage of peak flow), resulting in a stable insufflation flow at the end of inspiration. This stable flow corresponds to the leak flow rate. In consequence, the insufflation time will be prolonged and cycling delayed, which is very uncomfortable for the patient. In this case, the time cycle backup for the pressure support breath terminates inspiration.

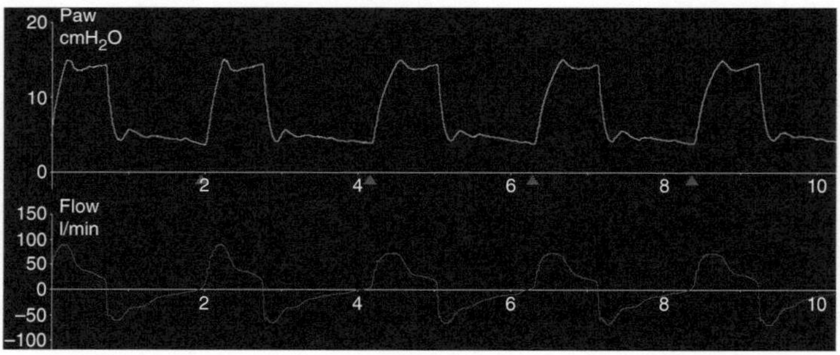

Leaks during insufflation:

1. Shorten the inspiratory time
2. Induce a more rapid decline in flow
3. Delay cycling
4. Improve patient-ventilator synchrony
5. May be indicated by a fast flow decay at the end of insufflation

5.11 Inspiratory Flow Distortion

A *change in the slope of the flow*'s exponential decline means a change in compliance or patient effort. If the slope of the flow flattens, this indicates inspiratory muscle relaxation. Conversely, if the slope of the flow becomes steeper, this indicates either a decrease in lung compliance (beginning of lung overdistension) or the start of an active expiratory effort.

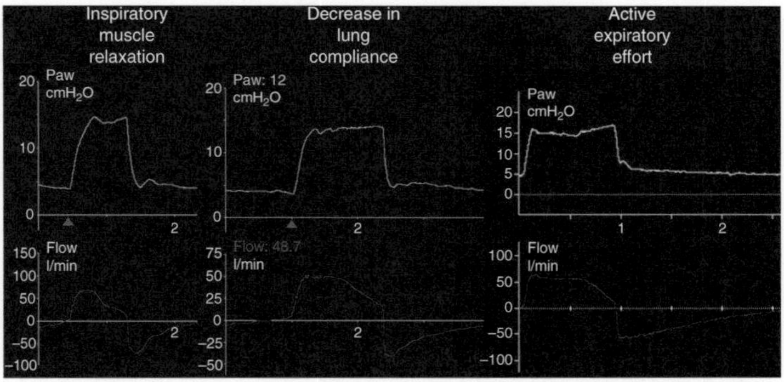

All statements regarding the flow during insufflation are true *except*:

1. Flow normally demonstrates an exponential decline
2. Flow slope may change in the case of lung overdistension
3. Flow may be linear
4. Flow slope is dependent on the inspiratory time constant
5. Flow slope may change in the case of active expiration

5.12 Early Cycling

Early cycling typically occurs when the *patient's inspiratory effort is prolonged past the end of the cycle event*. In pressure support, this is rare but could be caused by a flow cycle threshold set too high. As a consequence, the airway pressure will fall to below PEEP at the beginning of expiration. Simultaneously, the peak expiratory flow is reduced and followed by a short deviation of the flow toward the baseline (upward convexity), indicating a continued inspiratory effort even as pressure stored in the lungs is causing expiratory flow. The decline in expiratory flow has a normal shape when the inspiratory effort stops.

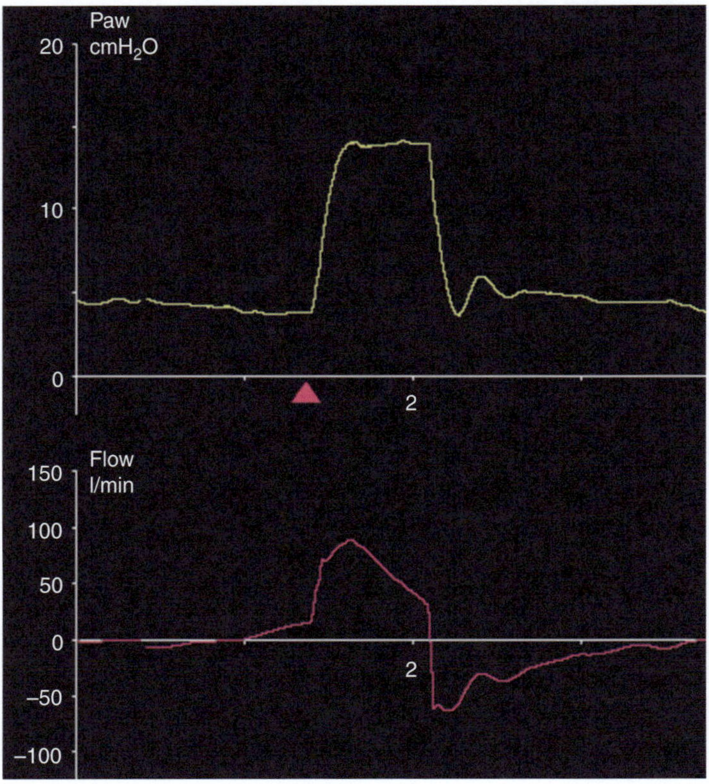

Early cycling is demonstrated by:

1. A long insufflation time
2. A rise in pressure at the end of inspiration
3. An increase in the peak expiratory flow
4. The absence of expiratory flow
5. A short deviation of the flow toward the baseline immediately after the peak in expiratory flow

5.13 Delayed Cycling

Delayed cycling typically occurs when the *patient's inspiratory ceases before the cycle threshold is met*. In pressure support, this may occur if the cycle threshold is set too low. The airway pressure shows a small increase above the set pressure at the end of insufflation. Simultaneously, the slope of the inspiratory flow becomes steeper.

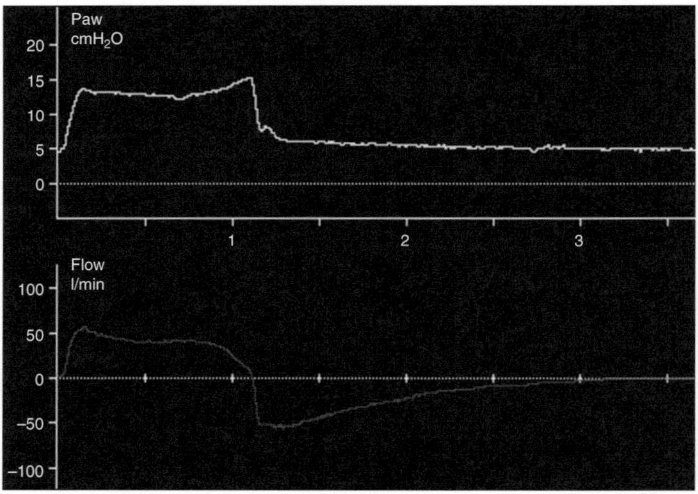

Delayed cycling is demonstrated by all these *except*:

1. A long insufflation time
2. A rise in airway pressure at the end of insufflation
3. Patient discomfort
4. A change of flow slope at the end of insufflation
5. Continuance of a stable flow at the end of insufflation

5.14 Delayed Cycling and Patient Inspiratory Effort

Delayed cycling and the relaxation of a strong inspiratory effort are both indicated by a *rise in pressure at the end of insufflation*. The shape of the inspiratory flow helps us to determine the cause. In the case of a strong inspiratory effort, the inspiratory flow has a rounded shape. In the case of delayed cycling, the inspiratory flow has a normal triangular shape or a stable flow at the end of insufflation where unintentional leaks are the cause of the delayed cycling.

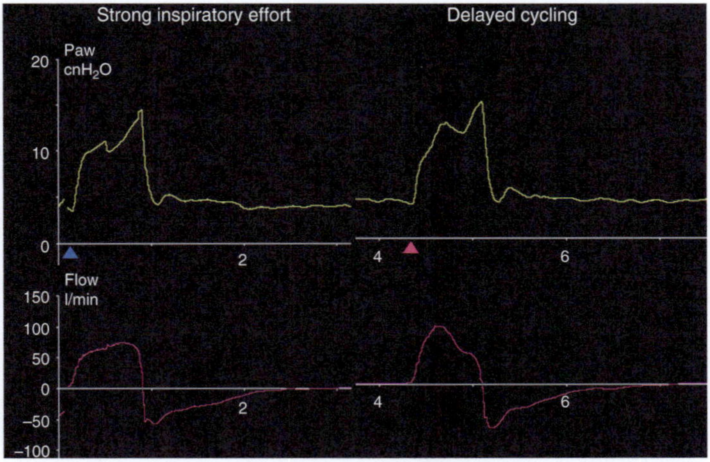

Delayed cycling and patient inspiratory effort can be determined:

1. By observing the pressure curve during insufflation
2. By observing the pressure curve during expiration
3. From the shape of the inspiratory flow
4. From the shape of the expiratory flow
5. By changing the inspiratory trigger sensitivity

5.15 Upper Airway Obstruction

Peak inspiratory flow is determined by the driving pressure (pressure support level above PEEP plus inspiratory effort) and inspiratory resistance. Peak expiratory flow is determined by driving pressure (tidal volume divided by compliance, plus any expiratory effort) and expiratory resistance, which is typically higher than inspiratory resistance. A breath-by-breath decrease in both the peak inspiratory and peak expiratory flows occurs in the case of resistance changes such as upper airway obstruction. The upper airways may be unstable or may even collapse during sleep in obese patients. The decrease in flow is followed by a hypopnea (small flow) or an apnea (no flow) event. The event ends with a micro-arousal that opens the upper airways again with a high peak inspiratory and expiratory flow.

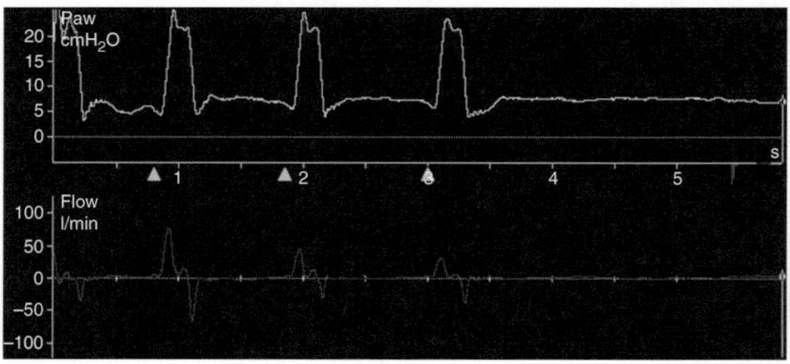

All statements regarding upper airway obstruction are true *except*:

1. Upper airway obstruction is demonstrated by a rapid decrease in the peak inspiratory and expiratory flows
2. Upper airway obstruction is demonstrated by a decrease in inspiratory flow only
3. Upper airway obstruction increases resistance
4. Upper airway obstruction induces hypopnea or apnea
5. Upper airway obstruction terminates with a micro-arousal

5.16 Cheyne-Stokes Respiration

Cheyne-Stokes respiration is an *oscillation of ventilation* between progressively deeper and sometimes faster breathing (hyperpnea) and a gradual decrease that results in a temporary stop in breathing (apnea). The pattern repeats itself in a cycle usually taking 30 s to 2 min. This abnormal pattern of breathing is caused by damage to respiratory centers (e.g., stroke) or physiological abnormalities associated with chronic heart failure.

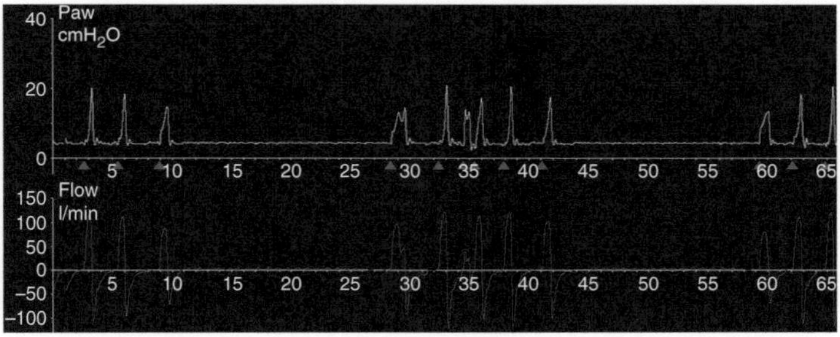

All statements regarding Cheyne-Stokes respiration are true *except*:

1. Cheyne-Stokes respiration is demonstrated on the pressure curve
2. Cheyne-Stokes respiration is demonstrated on the flow curve
3. Cheyne-Stokes respiration is a cause of central apnea
4. Cheyne-Stokes respiration occurs only during sleep
5. Cheyne-Stokes respiration can occur in healthy subject during sleep at high altitude

Responses

5.1 3

5.2 3

Answers 1, 2, 4, and 5 are true but not specific of unintentional leaks

5.3 1

5. This means that there is a leak on the expiratory valve

5.4 3

5.5 3

5.6 4

5.7 1

5.8 2

5.9 2

5.10 3

5.11 3

5.12 5

5.13 5

5.14 3

5.15 2

5.16 4

Suggested Readings

Carlucci A, Pisani L, et al. Patient-ventilator asynchronies: may the respiratory mechanics play a role? Crit Care. 2013;17(2):R54.

Carteaux G, Lyazidi A, et al. Patient-ventilator asynchrony during noninvasive ventilation: a bench and clinical study. Chest. 2012;142:367–76.

Hess DR. Ventilator waveforms and the physiology of pressure support ventilation. Respir Care. 2005;50:166–86.

Hess DR. Patient-ventilator interaction during noninvasive ventilation. Respir Care. 2011;56:153–65.

Vignaux L, Vargas F, et al. Patient-ventilator asynchrony during noninvasive ventilation for acute respiratory failure: a multicenter study. Intensive Care Med. 2009;35:840–6.

Chapter 6
Pressure-Volume Loop

6.1 Quasi-Static Pressure-Volume Loop

A quasi-static pressure-volume (PV) loop is a diagnostic maneuver used to assess the *elastic properties* of the respiratory system at each level of pressure during inflation and deflation of the lung. With the patient completely passive, either a low constant flow or slow pressure ramp is used to inflate the lungs from 0 up to 40 cm H_2O and then decreased gradually from 40 down to 0 cm H_2O. The slope of the PV loop at each point of pressure represents the compliance of the respiratory system (Video 6.1).

Electronic Supplementary Material The online version of this chapter (https://doi.org/10.1007/978-3-319-58655-7_6) contains supplementary material, which is available to authorized users.

J.-M. Arnal, *Monitoring Mechanical Ventilation Using Ventilator Waveforms*, https://doi.org/10.1007/978-3-319-58655-7_6

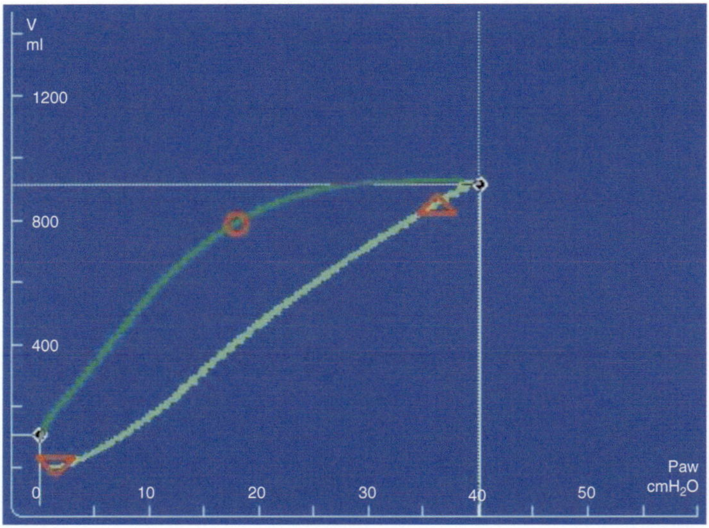

All statements regarding quasi-static PV loop are true *except*:

1. Can be performed at any level of pressure
2. Requires a low flow
3. Is a diagnostic maneuver
4. Provides information about resistance
5. Provides information about compliance at each level of pressure

6.2 Flow When Performing the PV Loop

In order to assess the elastic properties of the respiratory system only, the inflation and deflation flows *should be less than 10 l/min*. If the flow is higher, the resistive component will cause the PV loop to shift to the right (higher pressure). Prior to interpretation, the reliability of the PV loop should therefore be checked by displaying the flow-pressure loop.

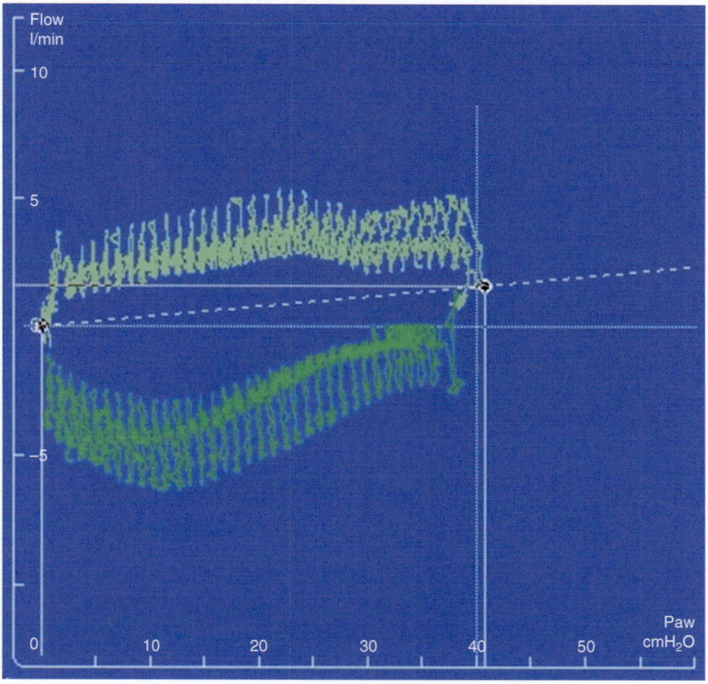

When performing a PV loop, the flow:

1. May affect the shape of the loop
2. May shift the loop on the X-axis
3. Should be less than 10 l/min
4. Depends on the compliance
5. All are true

6.3 PV Loop in a Normal Lung

In a normal lung that is fully aerated at the beginning of the maneuver, the pressure-volume relation is linear. This means that *compliance remains constant* throughout inflation. Deflation is also linear. There is a small degree of physiological hysteresis (area between the inflation and deflation limbs of the PV loop) that occurs due to the viscoelastic property of tissues.

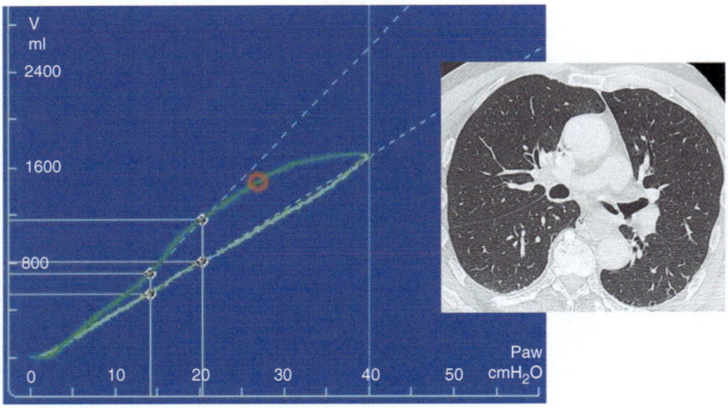

A low-flow PV loop in a normal lung shows:

1. A large degree of hysteresis
2. A change in the slope during deflation
3. A linear inflation limb and a small degree of hysteresis
4. A change in the slope during inflation
5. The same loop as a dynamic PV loop

6.4 PV Loop in ARDS

In an early-onset ARDS patient, the shape of the PV loop may differ compared to that of a normal-lung patient. The inflation and deflation limbs demonstrate a *change in slope*, which means that the respiratory-system compliance varies at different levels of pressure. In addition, *hysteresis* is greater than in normal-lung patients due to recruitment occurring during inflation and derecruitment occurring during deflation. Therefore, a quasi-static PV loop can be used to assess the potential for recruitment and predict the effect of a recruitment maneuver.

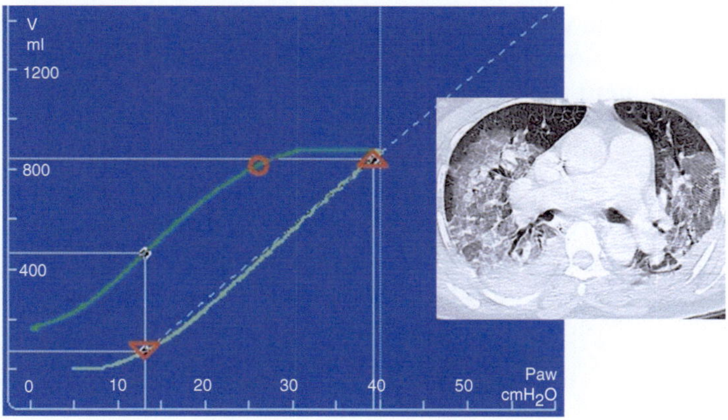

A PV loop in an ARDS patient is used to:

1. Determine the optimal PEEP setting
2. Assess the lung recruitability
3. Predict the effect of a recruitment maneuver
4. Determine the compliance at each level of pressure
5. All but one

6.5 Change in Slope During Inflation

In an early-onset ARDS patient, recruitment takes place throughout inflation. At the beginning of inflation, the slope is almost horizontal (low compliance) because the gas inflates partially collapsed lung. Compliance is low due to the small volume of aerated lung (baby lung). Subsequently, there is a change in the slope that is incorrectly referred to as the *low inflection point*. It is more correctly called the point of “maximum curvature” or “maximum compliance change.” The inflection point is where compliance goes from increasing to decreasing and occurs about midway up the curve. From the lower point of maximum curvature onward, the volume increases more for the same increase in pressure (slowly increasing compliance). This is due to lung recruitment with popping open of collapsed alveoli. Sometimes there is another change in the slope at a high inflation pressure that is incorrectly referred to as the upper inflection point. Rather, this is the upper point of maximum curvature. Above this point, very little recruitment takes place, and all the gas inflates the already aerated lung. When the last part of the loop flattens, this means there is lung overdistension. Maximum recruitment therefore occurs in the range of pressure between the two points of maximum curvature.

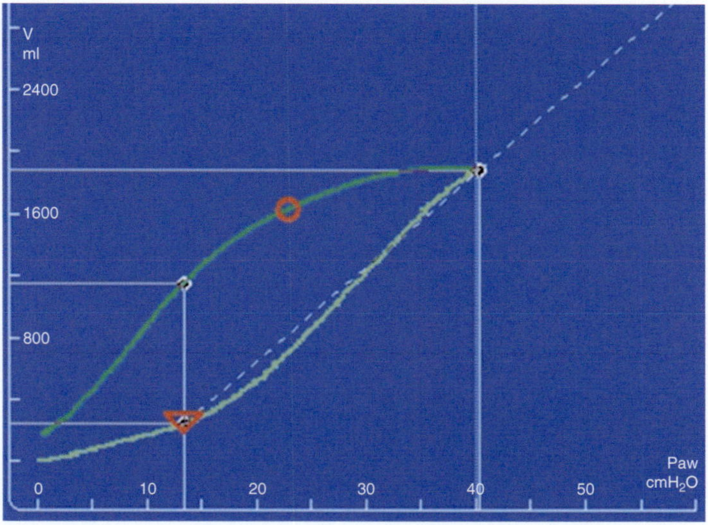

The inflation limb of the PV loop demonstrates:

1. Low compliance at a low inflation pressure due to the baby lung
2. A change in slope in recruiters
3. A linear increase in non-recruiters
4. Lung overdistension at high inflation pressure
5. All are true

6.6 Linear Compliance

Linear compliance or midrange compliance is the compliance of the recruiting part of the inflation limb, i.e., *between the two changes in the slope*. The more vertical the slope, the more recruitment takes place. Therefore, high linear compliance equates to high potential for recruitment. Linear compliance is different to static compliance. As a general rule, it can be said that if the linear compliance is double the static compliance, there is high potential for recruitment.

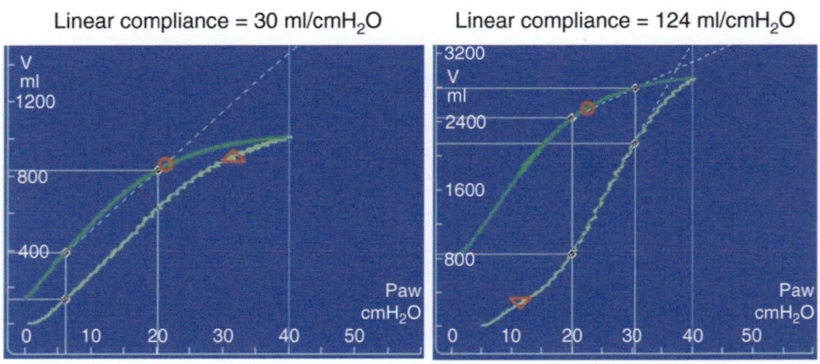

All statements regarding linear compliance are true *except*:

1. Linear compliance is measured from 0 to 40 cmH_2O
2. Linear compliance indicates the potential for lung recruitment
3. Linear compliance is higher than static compliance in recruiters
4. Linear compliance is close to static compliance in non-recruiters
5. Linear compliance is measured between the two changes in slope during inflation

6.7 Chest-Wall Effect

If there is a load on the chest wall, the *first part of the inflation limb may be flat* with no volume increase. Volume increase starts at the level of pressure where the chest-wall pressure has been overcome. This phenomenon occurs in the case of increased abdominal pressure, severe obesity, abundant edema, etc.

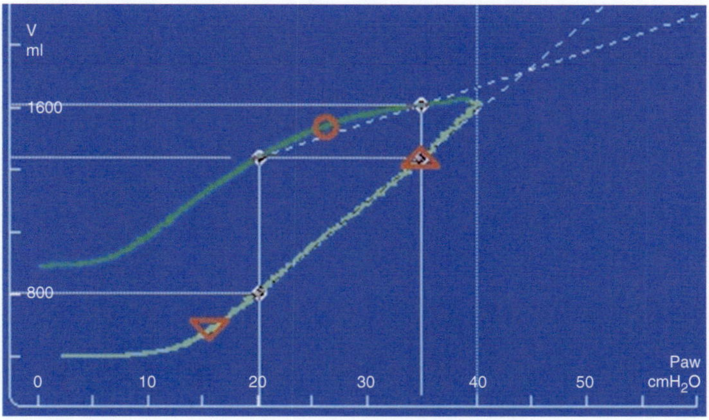

Which of the statements is not true? In case of a heavy chest wall:

1. The lung is usually recruitable
2. The first part of inflation is flat with no volume increase
3. There is no change in the inflation slope
4. A higher pressure is needed to recruit the lung
5. A higher PEEP is required to keep the lung aerated

6.8 Change in Slope During Deflation

Derecruitment is a continuous process that occurs throughout deflation. The deflation limb is almost flat at the beginning of deflation, which means that there is little or no derecruitment at high pressure. Subsequently, the slope of the deflation limb changes at a point referred to as the deflection point or *point of maximum curvature* during deflation. The deflection point is usually located somewhere above 20 cmH_2O of pressure. Below this point, deflation and derecruitment occur. The slope of deflation usually remains linear from this point down to baseline pressure. In patients with high potential for recruitment, the volume at the end of deflation is greater than zero. This means that all the volume recruited during inflation was not entirely derecruited during deflation. Therefore, the functional residual capacity is higher after the maneuver than before.

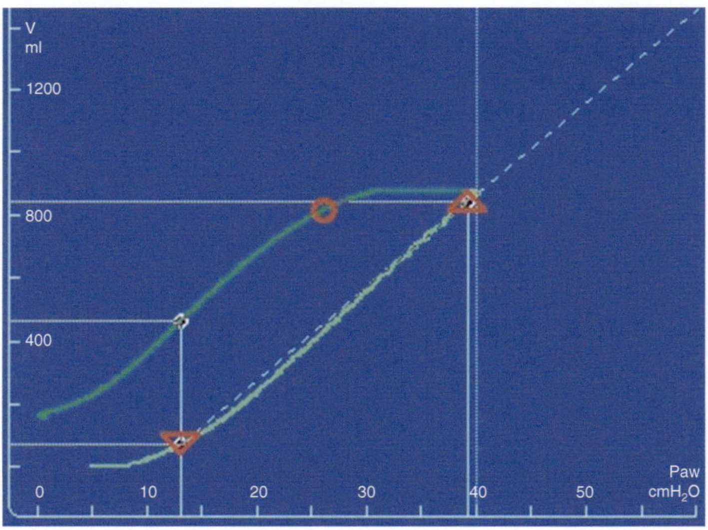

The deflation limb of the PV loop:

1. Is usually linear
2. Demonstrates a change in slope at high pressure
3. Shows that derecruitment and deflation occur at the different pressures
4. May help to assess lung recruitability
5. Returns to the same baseline volume if recruitment occurred during the maneuver

6.9 Hysteresis

Hysteresis is the *area between the inflation and deflation limbs* of the PV loop. In an ARDS patient, hysteresis may be much greater than in a normal-lung patient due to recruitment occurring during inflation and derecruitment occurring during deflation. Recruitment occurs at a higher pressure than derecruitment. Therefore, the volume of the respiratory system at any given pressure is higher during deflation than during inflation. The larger the volume difference between inflation and deflation, the higher the potential for recruitment. Hysteresis is quite awkward to calculate but can easily be estimated using the volume difference between inflation and deflation measured at 20 cm H_2O of pressure. If the volume difference is higher than 500 ml, it means there is high potential for recruitment.

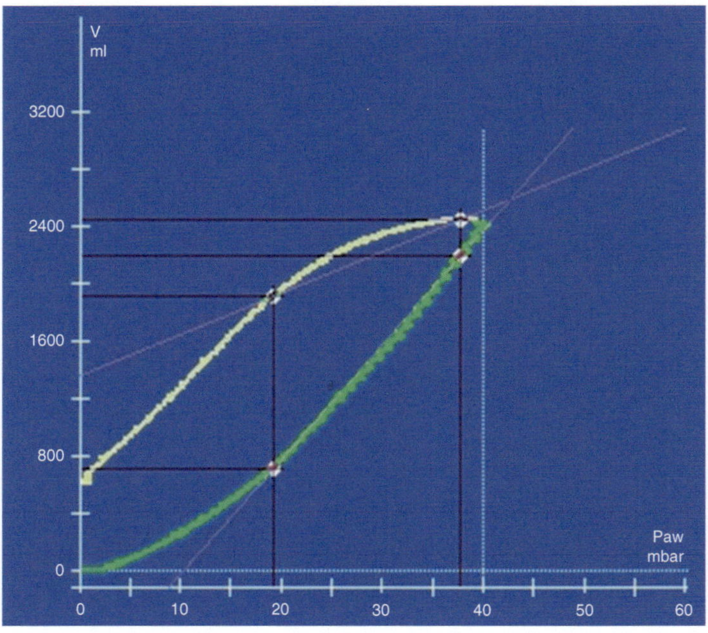

All statements regarding hysteresis are true *except*:

1. Hysteresis is the volume difference between the inflation and deflation limbs
2. Hysteresis is the area between the inflation and deflation limbs
3. Hysteresis is greater in patients with high potential for recruitment
4. Hysteresis is mainly due to recruitment during inflation and derecruitment during deflation in ARDS patients
5. Hysteresis can be estimated as the volume difference between inflation and deflation at 20 cmH_2O

6.10 Hysteresis in COPD

Hysteresis can be considerable in COPD patients for reasons other than recruitment/derecruitment. COPD patients have *lung emphysema and lung heterogeneity* with long time-constant bronchoalveoli, which are slow to inflate and deflate. Therefore, a low-flow PV loop is not of any value in an ARDS patient with COPD. In addition, it is not recommended to increase pressure to 40 cm H_2O due to the risk of volutrauma.

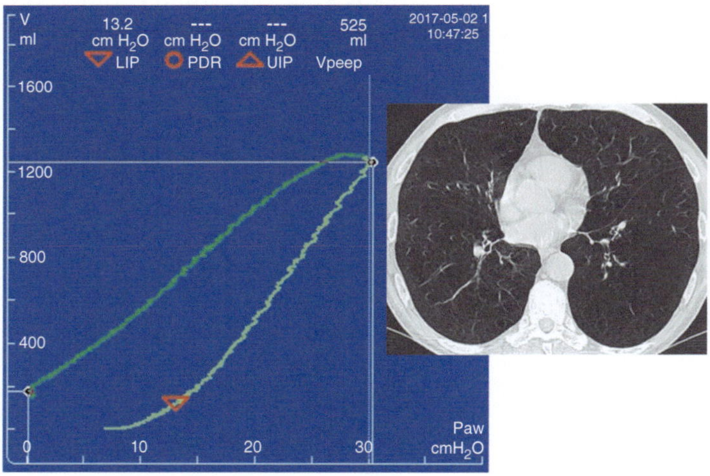

In COPD patients, hysteresis:

1. Has the same meaning as in ARDS
2. Is usually absent
3. Is used to assess the potential for lung recruitment
4. Is mainly due to long time-constant bronchoalveoli
5. Should be considered to set PEEP

6.11 Assessing the Potential for Recruitment

A quasi-static PV loop is *mainly used in ARDS patients to assess the potential for recruitment* and predict the efficacy of a recruitment maneuver. Patients with high potential for recruitment demonstrate a change in slope on the inflation limb, a high linear (midrange) compliance, and a large degree of hysteresis. Conversely, patients with low potential for recruitment demonstrate a linear inflation limb, a low linear compliance, and a small degree of hysteresis (Videos 6.2 and 6.3).

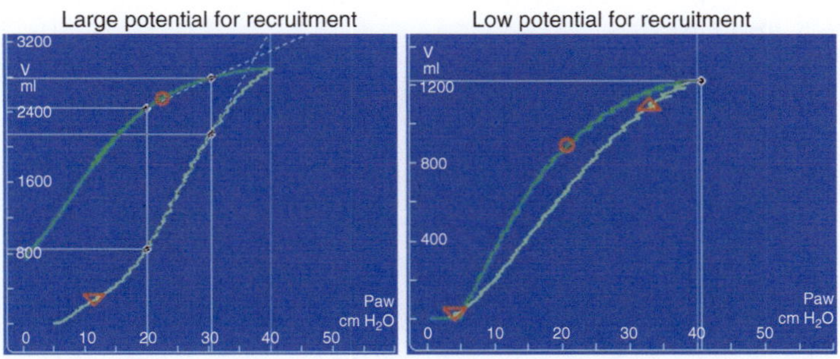

The quasi-static PV loop for a patient with high recruitment potential shows:

1. A point of increase on the inflation slope
2. Sometimes a point of decrease on the inflation slope
3. Linear compliance that is double the static compliance
4. A large degree of hysteresis
5. All of the above

6.12 Recruitment Maneuvers

If the user sets a pause at the highest pressure of the PV loop (when the quasi-static PV curve is generated with a pressure ramp), this serves as a *sustained inflation recruitment maneuver* that can be used to re-inflate the collapsed lung. This maneuver should only be performed in patients with high potential for recruitment and with no contraindications. The volume increase at the highest pressure is an assessment of the volume of the collapsed lung that was re-inflated, assuming there is no leakage from the ventilator circuit (Videos 6.4, 6.5, and 6.6).

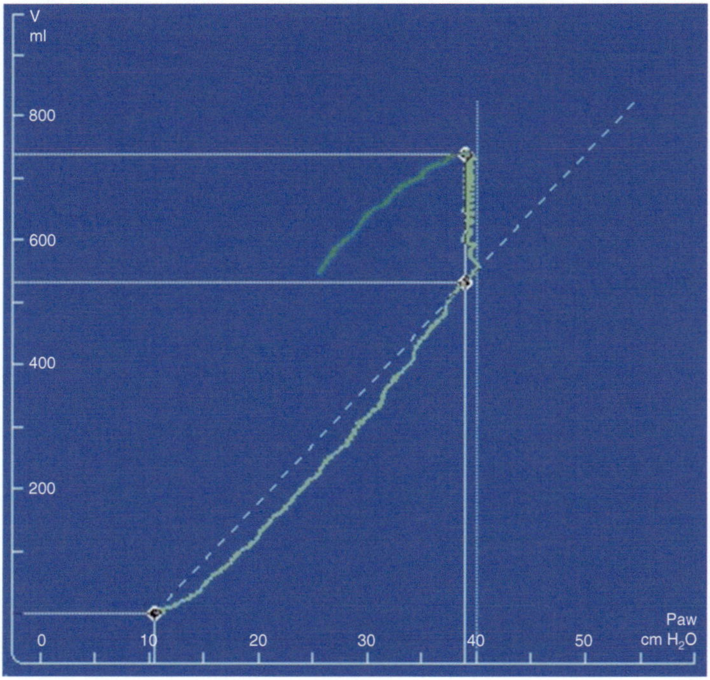

All statements are true except one. The quasi-static PV loop can be used as a sustained inflation recruitment maneuver:

1. By setting a pause at the highest pressure
2. In patients with high potential of recruitment
3. In the absence of contraindications
4. With the possibility of monitoring the volume recruited
5. With the possibility of monitoring hysteresis

Responses

6.1 4

6.2 5

3. Nowadays ventilator offers PV loop tool. In some of them, user set the flow and the range of pressure. Therefore, duration of the maneuver depends on the compliance. In some of them, user has to set the pressure ramp (e.g., 2 cm H_2O per second) and the range of pressure. Therefore duration of the maneuver is constant, but flow varies at each step according to compliance.

6.3 3

6.4 5

6.5 5

6.6 1

6.7 3

6.8 2

6.9 1

6.10 4

6.11 5

6.12 5

Suggested Readings

Albaiceta GM, Taboada F, et al. Tomographic study of the inflection points of the pressure-volume curve in acute lung injury. Am J Respir Crit Care Med. 2004;170:1066–72.

Bachofen H. Lung tissue resistance and pulmonary hysteresis. J Appl Physiol. 1968;24:296–301.

Chiumello D, Carlesso E, et al. Effects of volume shift on the pressure-volume curve of the respiratory system in ALI/ARDS patients. Minerva Anestesiol. 2007;73:109–18.

Crotti S, Mascheroni D, et al. Recruitment and derecruitment during acute respiratory failure: a clinical study. Am J Respir Crit Care Med. 2001;164:131–40.

Decailliot F, Demoule A, et al. Pressure-volume curves with and without muscle paralysis in acute respiratory distress syndrome. Intensive Care Med. 2006;32:1322–8.

Demory D, Arnal JM, et al. Recruitability of the lung estimated by the pressure volume curve hysteresis in ARDS patients. Intensive Care Med. 2008;34:2019–25.

DiRocco JD, Carney DE, et al. Correlation between alveolar recruitment/derecruitment and inflection points on the pressure-volume curve. Intensive Care Med. 2007;33:1204–11.

Gattinoni L, Mascheroni D, et al. Volume/pressure curve of total respiratory system in paralysed patients: artefacts and correction factors. Intensive Care Med. 1987;13:19–25.

Gattinoni L, Caironi P, et al. Lung recruitment in patients with the acute respiratory distress syndrome. N Engl J Med. 2006;354:1775–86.

Harris RS. Pressure-volume curves of the respiratory system. Respir Care. 2005;50:78–98.

Harris RS, Hess DR, et al. An objective analysis of the pressure-volume curve in the acute respiratory distress syndrome. Am J Respir Crit Care Med. 2000;161:432–9.

Hickling KG. The pressure-volume curve is greatly modified by recruitment. A mathematical model of ARDS lungs. Am J Respir Crit Care Med. 1998;158:194–202.

Hickling KG. Best compliance during a decremental, but not incremental, positive end-expiratory pressure trial is related to open-lung positive end-expiratory pressure: a mathematical model of acute respiratory distress syndrome lungs. Am J Respir Crit Care Med. 2001;163:69–78.

Hickling KG. Reinterpreting the pressure-volume curve in patients with acute respiratory distress syndrome. Curr Opin Crit Care. 2002;8:32–8.

Jonson B. Elastic pressure-volume curves in acute lung injury and acute respiratory distress syndrome. Intensive Care Med. 2005;31:205–12.

Jonson B, Richard JC, et al. Pressure-volume curves and compliance in acute lung injury: evidence of recruitment above the lower inflection point. Am J Respir Crit Care Med. 1999;159:1172–8.

Maggiore SM, Brochard L. Pressure-volume curve: methods and meaning. Minerva Anestesiol. 2001;67:228–37.

Maggiore SM, Jonson B, et al. Alveolar derecruitment at decremental positive end-expiratory pressure levels in acute lung injury: comparison with the lower inflection point, oxygenation, and compliance. Am J Respir Crit Care Med. 2001;164:795–801.

Maggiore SM, Richard JC, et al. What has been learnt from P/V curves in patients with acute lung injury/acute respiratory distress syndrome. Eur Respir J Suppl. 2003;42:22s–6s.

Matamis D, Lemaire F, et al. Total respiratory pressure-volume curves in the adult respiratory distress syndrome. Chest. 1984;86:58–66.

Ranieri VM, Brienza N, et al. Impairment of lung and chest wall mechanics in patients with acute respiratory distress syndrome: role of abdominal distension. Am J Respir Crit Care Med. 1997;156:1082–91.

Servillo G, De Robertis E, et al. The upper inflection point of the pressure-volume curve. Influence of methodology and of different modes of ventilation. Intensive Care Med. 2002;28:842–9.

Thille AW, Richard JC, et al. Alveolar recruitment in pulmonary and extrapulmonary acute respiratory distress syndrome: comparison using pressure-volume curve or static compliance. Anesthesiology. 2007;106:212–7.

Venegas JG, Harris RS, et al. A comprehensive equation for the pulmonary pressure-volume curve. J Appl Physiol. 1998;84:389–95.

Chapter 7
Esophageal Pressure Curve

7.1 The Esophageal Pressure Curve in Passive Patients

7.1.1 Normal Curve

Esophageal pressure (P_{ES}) is measured by a balloon inflated with air, positioned in the lower third of the esophagus *in order to estimate pleural pressure*. In a passive patient, esophageal pressure increases with each mechanical insufflation. Small, rapid oscillations come from the heart and pulmonary circulation. Transpulmonary pressure (P_{TP}) is calculated as airway pressure (P_{AW}) minus P_{ES} (Video 7.1).

Electronic Supplementary Material The online version of this chapter (https://doi.org/10.1007/978-3-319-58655-7_7) contains supplementary material, which is available to authorized users.

J.-M. Arnal, *Monitoring Mechanical Ventilation Using Ventilator Waveforms*, https://doi.org/10.1007/978-3-319-58655-7_7

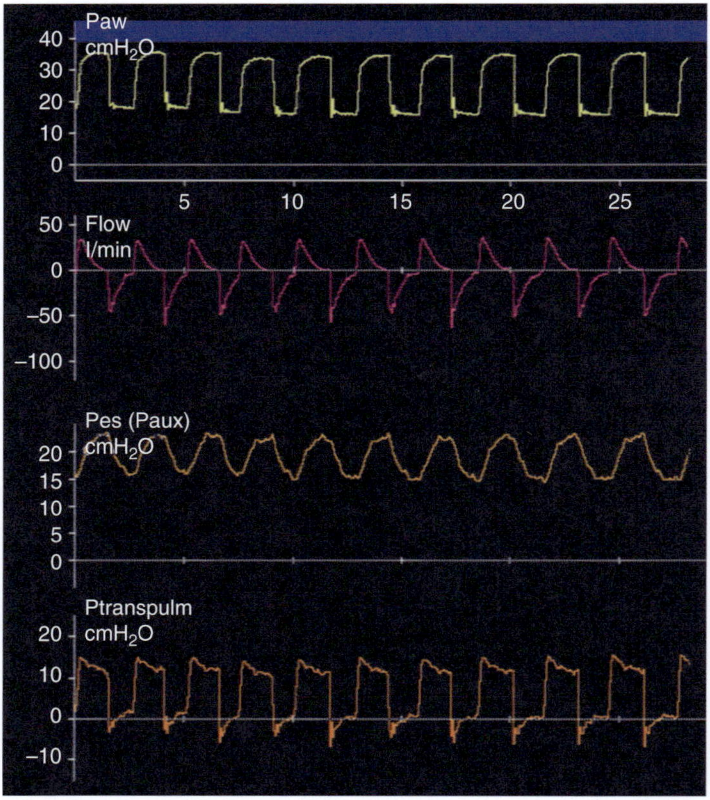

All statements regarding P_{ES} in a passive patient are true *except*:

1. P_{ES} is always positive
2. P_{ES} increases during insufflation
3. P_{ES} decreases at the beginning of inspiration
4. P_{ES} is measured at the lower third in the esophagus
5. P_{ES} is used to calculate transpulmonary pressure

7.1.2 Positioning

The esophageal balloon is firstly inserted into the stomach and inflated. The stomach pressure curve shows a low baseline with a small positive swing during insufflation. Gentle pressure on the stomach will then increase the pressure. Subsequently, the catheter is slowly pulled out until the point where *cardiogenic oscillations appear*. (Video 7.2).

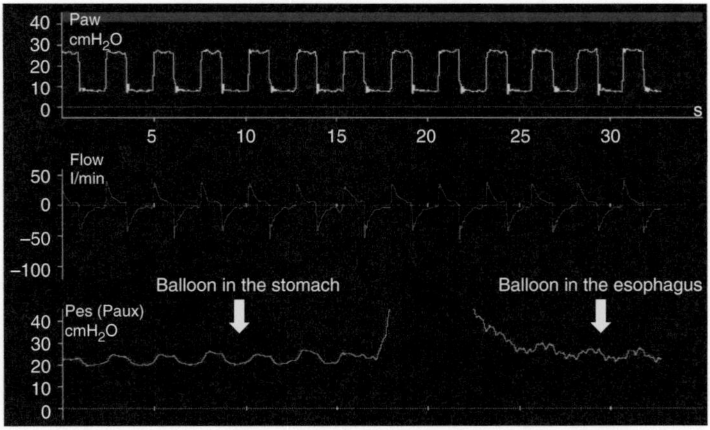

The balloon is positioned in the lower third of the esophagus if:

1. There is a positive swing during insufflation
2. Cardiogenic oscillations can be seen
3. The pressure during expiration is above baseline
4. The pressure increases when the stomach is pressed
5. The pressure curve is similar to the airway pressure curve

7.1.3 Occlusion Test in Passive Patient

An occlusion test can be used to check the correct positioning of the esophageal balloon. An end-expiratory occlusion is performed. The clinician presses gently with both hands symmetrically on the chest for a couple of seconds and then releases the pressure. P_{AW} and P_{ES} increase simultaneously during the manual pressure. The positioning is correct if the *increase in* P_{AW} *and* P_{ES} *is the same*, i.e., transpulmonary pressure remains stable during the occlusion test (Video 7.3).

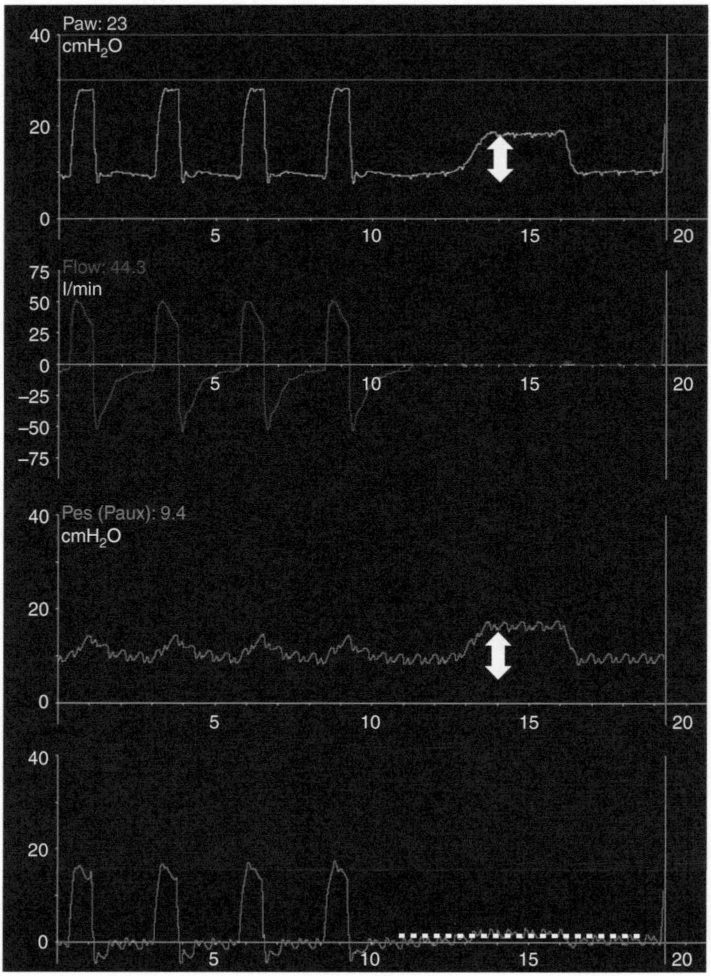

During the occlusion test:

1. Manual pressure on the chest increases P_{AW}
2. Manual pressure on the chest decreases P_{ES}
3. Transpulmonary pressure remains stable if the balloon is positioned correctly
4. There is no flow
5. All of the above

7.1.4 Inflation of the Esophageal Balloon

After optimal placement, optimal inflation of the esophageal balloon is tested by gradually filling the balloon in increments of 0.5 ml for small-volume balloons and 1 ml for large-volume balloons, while simultaneously measuring the esophageal pressure. The *optimal volume is the one associated with the largest tidal increase in* P_{ES} (Video 7.4).

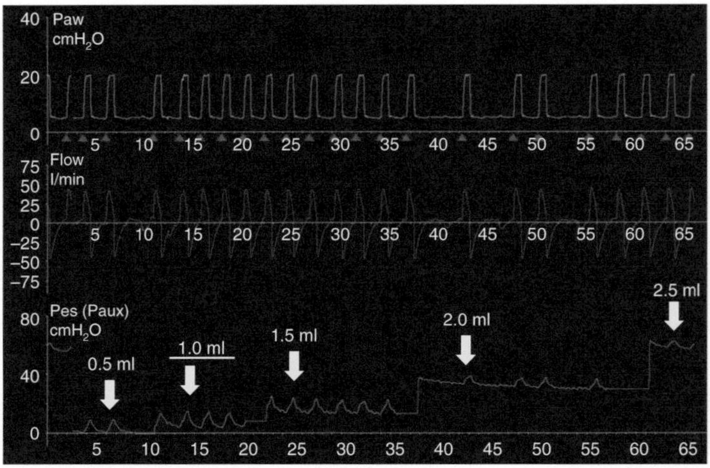

All statements are true except one. The optimal filling volume for an esophageal balloon:

1. Is always the same
2. Depends on esophageal wall compliance
3. Is tested for each patient
4. Differs depending on the catheter used
5. Affects the measurement of esophageal pressure

7.1.5 Transalveolar Pressure

Transalveolar pressure (P_{TA}) is the elastic recoil pressure of the lung, calculated as *alveolar pressure minus P_{ES}*. P_{TA} is often calculated using P_A and P_{ES} at end inspiration and end expiration by means of end-inspiratory and end-expiratory occlusions, respectively (when alveolar pressure, P_A, equals airway pressure, P_{AW}). During occlusions, flow is zero and $P_{TA} = P_{TP}$. P_{TA} is the pressure that recruits the lung during insufflation or a recruitment maneuver and keeps the lung inflated at end expiration. It also has the potential to injure the lung (increased strain, because ΔV = elastance × ΔP_{TA}). P_{TA} is an important variable to monitor in passive ARDS patients, to enable the application of an open-lung strategy and help prevent lung injuries.

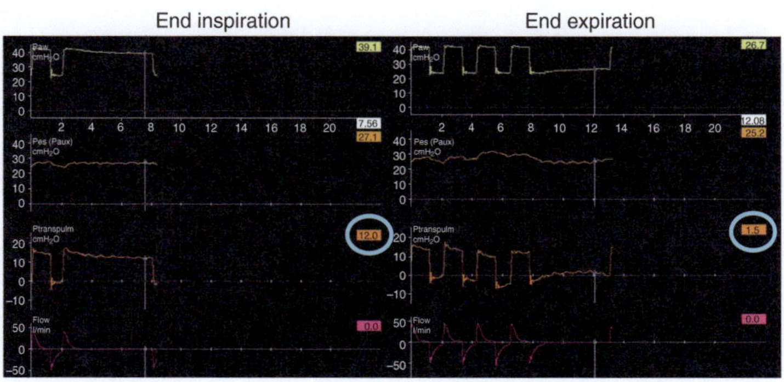

All statements regarding transalveolar pressure are true *except*:

1. P_{TA} is calculated as P_{AW} minus P_{ES}
2. P_{TA} is calculated at end inspiration as P_{PLAT} minus P_{ES}
3. P_{TA} can't be monitored continuously
4. P_{TA} represents the stress applied to the lung
5. P_{TA} is calculated at end expiration as $PEEP_{TOT}$ minus P_{ES}

7.1.6 P_{TA} at End Inspiration

P_{TA} at end inspiration is calculated as P_{PLAT} minus P_{ES} measured by means of a 5-s *end-inspiratory occlusion*. P_{TA} at end inspiration represents the stress applied to the lung and should be limited to less than 15 cmH_2O

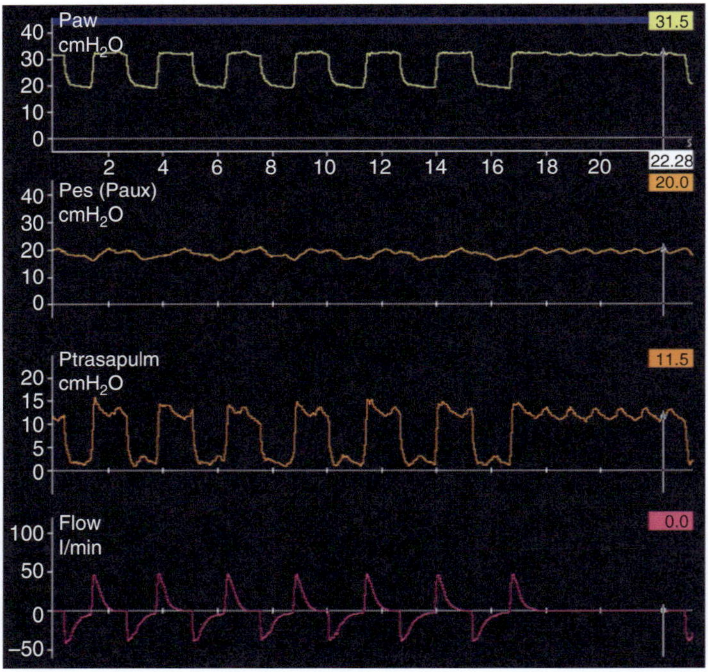

P_{TA} at end inspiration:

1. Is an assessment of the stress applied to the lung
2. Is an assessment of the strain applied to the lung
3. Should be limited to less than 25 cmH_2O
4. Can be measured continuously
5. Can be estimated from P_{PLAT} without esophageal pressure measurement

7.1.7 P_{TA} at End Expiration

P_{TA} at end expiration is calculated as $PEEP_{TOT}$ minus P_{ES} measured by means of an *end-expiratory occlusion*. P_{TA} at end expiration may sometimes be negative in passive ARDS patients, which means that the pressure surrounding the alveoli in the middle thorax zone is higher than the alveolar pressure. Alveoli may collapse at end expiration, causing atelectrauma. Therefore, PEEP should be adjusted to maintain a positive P_{TA} at end expiration and thus prevent the risk of atelectrauma (Videos 7.5 and 7.6).

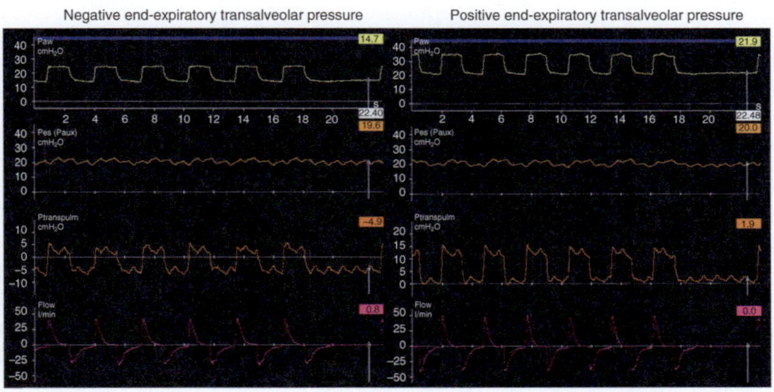

All statements regarding P_{TA} at end expiration are true *except*:

1. P_{TA} at end expiration is used to assess the risk of atelectrauma
2. P_{TA} at end expiration is used to set PEEP in passive ARDS patients
3. P_{TA} at end expiration is used to assess the middle thorax zone
4. P_{TA} at end expiration is used to assess the strain applied to the lung
5. P_{TA} at end expiration should be slightly positive

7.1.8 Transpulmonary Driving Pressure

Transpulmonary driving pressure (ΔP_{TA}) is the *elastic pressure required to inflate the lung with the tidal volume.* ΔP_{TA} is calculated as P_{TA} at end inspiration minus P_{TA} at end expiration and assesses the strain applied to the lung and is equal to V_T per unit of lung compliance. ΔP_{TA} is associated with clinical outcomes in ARDS patients and may be more closely associated with mortality than tidal volume per kg ideal body weight. Preliminary data suggests ΔP_{TA} should be maintained below 10 cm H_2O (Video 7.7).

$$\Delta P_L = P_{L\ end\text{-}ins} - P_{L\ end\text{-}exp} = 11 - 3 = 8\ cmH_2O$$

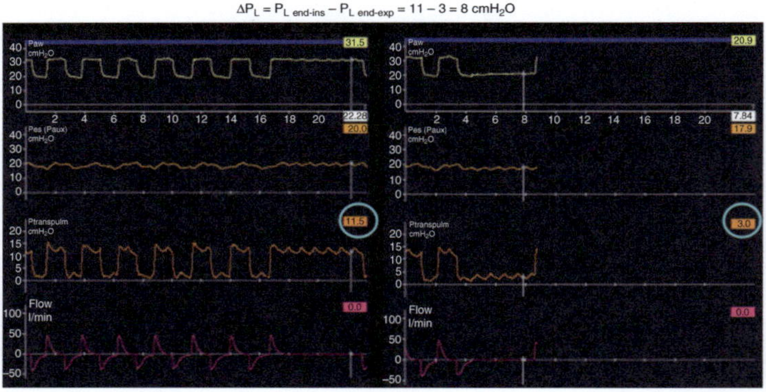

Transpulmonary driving pressure:

1. Should be kept below 10 cmH_2O
2. Can't be measured continuously
3. Is used to assess the strain applied to the lung
4. Can be used to set the tidal volume
5. All of the above

7.1.9 Transpulmonary Pressure-Volume Loop

A combination of esophageal pressure measurement and a quasi-static pressure-volume (PV) loop maneuver allows us to display a transpulmonary PV loop. This loop represents the PV loop of the lungs (i.e., separate from the chest wall) and is *more precise than an airway PV loop* for assessing the lung's recruitability (Videos 7.8 and 7.9).

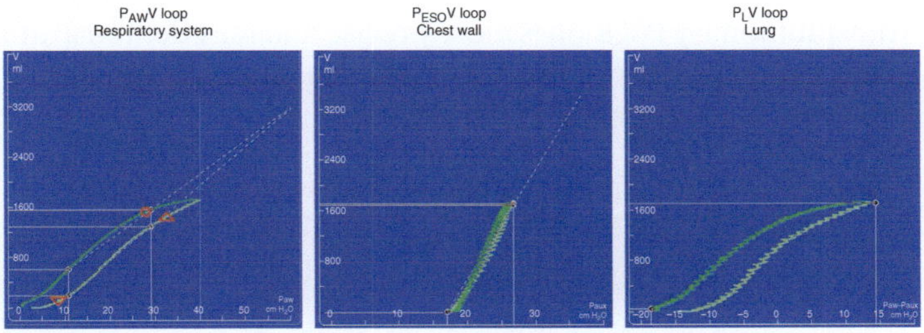

All statements regarding transpulmonary PV loop are true *except*:

1. Transpulmonary PV loop is similar to an airway PV loop
2. Transpulmonary PV loop plots transpulmonary pressure versus volume
3. Transpulmonary PV loop is independent of the chest-wall mechanics
4. Transpulmonary PV loop is used to assess lung recruitability
5. Transpulmonary PV loop is more precise than an airway PV loop

7.1.10 Airway and Transpulmonary PV Loops

In typical cases of high and low potential for lung recruitment, transrespiratory (i.e., P_{AW} minus pressure on the body surface) and transpulmonary PV loops show the same results in terms of the change in slope during inflation, linear compliance, and hysteresis. In some cases a transrespiratory PV loop is not informative because there *is no change in slope during inflation or linear compliance is not high*. In such cases, a transpulmonary PV loop is more precise and may demonstrate some potential for recruitment with a change in slope during inflation and higher linear compliance.

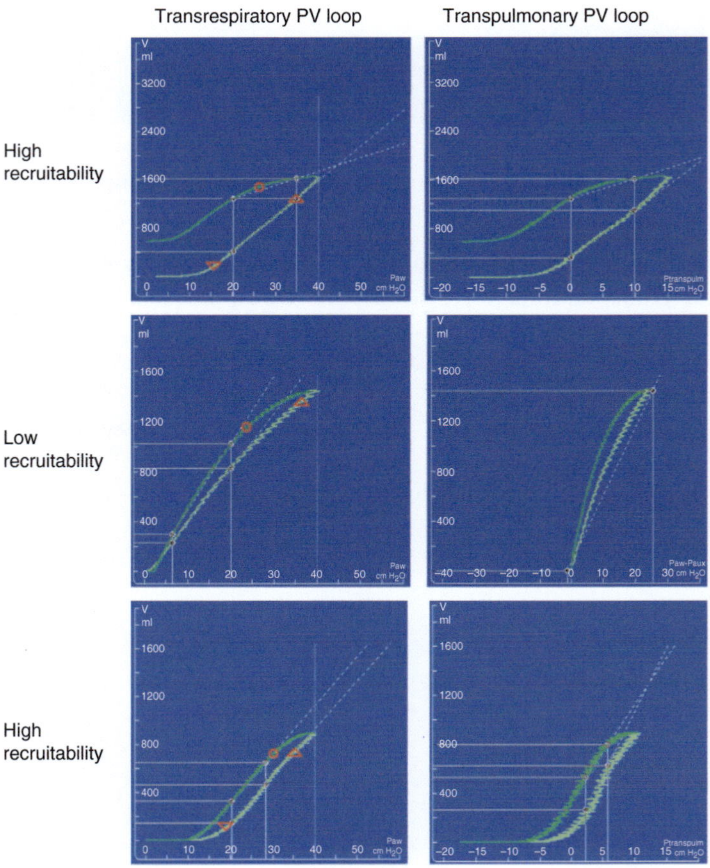

Transrespiratory and transpulmonary PV loops:

1. Have exactly the same shape
2. Display the same change in slope
3. Display the same linear compliance
4. Are measured with two successive maneuvers
5. Can have different shapes

7.1.11 Hysteresis

Hysteresis on the quasi-static transrespiratory PV loop is mainly due to recruitment during inflation and derecruitment during deflation. Consequently, there is *no hysteresis on the chest-wall PV loop* because there is no recruitment in the chest wall. The *entire hysteresis* measured on the transrespiratory PV loop is reproduced on the *transpulmonary PV loop*.

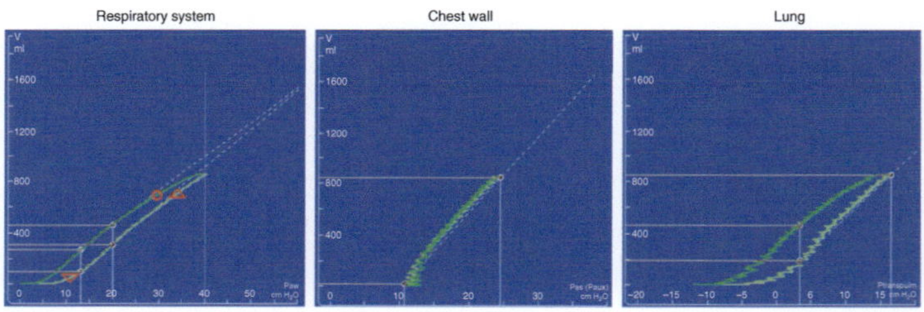

All statements regarding hysteresis are true *except*:

1. Hysteresis is seen on the transrespiratory PV loop
2. Hysteresis is explained by the chest-wall mechanics
3. Hysteresis is mainly due to recruitment and derecruitment of the lung
4. Hysteresis is seen on the transpulmonary pressure PV loop
5. Hysteresis is large in a patient with high potential for recruitment

7.1.12 Transpulmonary Pressure During Recruitment Maneuvers

A combination of esophageal pressure measurement and a sustained inflation recruitment maneuver allows us to monitor transpulmonary pressure during recruitment. *Transpulmonary pressure should be around 20 to 25 cmH$_2$O during a recruitment maneuver*, in order to reinflate the collapsed lung without injuring the lung. In some patients with high esophageal pressure, an airway pressure of up to 60 cmH$_2$O can be required to reach the target transpulmonary pressure during the recruitment maneuver (Video 7.10).

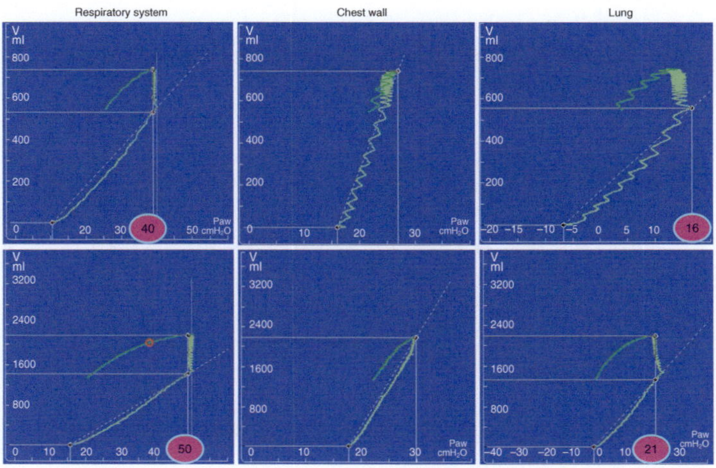

All statements are true except one. During a recruitment maneuver, transpulmonary pressure:

1. Is the pressure that reinflates the collapsed lung
2. Should be greater than the sum of surface tension and compressive pressures
3. Is dependent on chest-wall mechanics
4. Is seen on the transpulmonary recruitment maneuver loop
5. Helps to titrate the airway pressure required for recruitment

7.1.13 Increase in Volume During Recruitment Maneuvers

The volume increase during a sustained inflation recruitment maneuver is *mainly due to lung recruitment*. Because there is no recruitment in the chest wall, the chest-wall recruitment maneuver does not show any volume increase. Consequently, the entire volume increase seen in the respiratory-system recruitment maneuver is reproduced in the lung recruitment maneuver. In addition, *transpulmonary pressure decreases* during the recruitment maneuver. This is because the ventilator maintains a constant pressure at the airway opening, and esophageal pressure increases as lung volume increases. An increasing lung volume and decreasing transpulmonary pressure mean that lung compliance improves during the recruitment maneuver (Video 7.11).

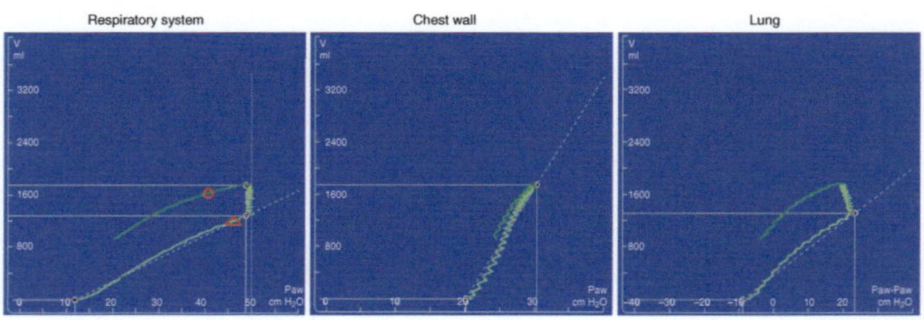

All statements are true except one. The volume increase during a recruitment maneuver:

1. Is overestimated in the case of leaks from the ventilator circuit
2. Is due to overdistension of the lung
3. Is an assessment of the volume of the lung that is reinflated
4. Is seen on the respiratory system and lung recruitment maneuver loops
5. Is associated with a gradual increase in lung compliance

7.1.14 Reverse Triggering

Reverse triggering occurs in highly sedated patients without paralysis, who are ventilated with ventilator triggered breaths. A reverse triggered breath is identified as having indications of an *inspiratory effort after the ventilator trigger event*. This may be observed as distortions of the pressure and/or the flow waveforms (or a negative esophageal pressure swing) starting at mid inspiration. Reverse triggering has clinical consequences, such as an increase in tidal volume and transpulmonary pressure, double triggering, an incorrect estimation of plateau pressure, etc. (Videos 7.12 and 7.13).

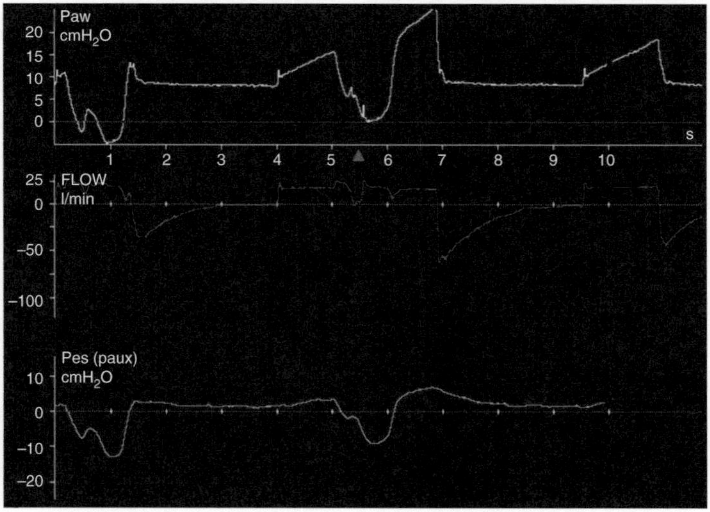

Reverse triggering:

1. Is a positive swing in esophageal pressure occurring during a ventilator triggered breath
2. Is a patient's inspiratory effort triggered by a ventilator triggered breath
3. Is a negative swing in esophageal pressure occurring near the end of a ventilator triggered breath
4. Is not clinically important
5. Both 2 and 3

7.2 Esophageal Pressure Curve in Spontaneously Breathing Patients

7.2.1 Normal Curve

In spontaneously breathing patients, P_{ES} *starts decreasing at the onset of the patient's inspiratory effort* and drops to a minimum pressure at the end of the inspiratory effort. Subsequently, P_{ES} increases up to baseline again during the relaxation phase (Videos 7.14 and 7.15).

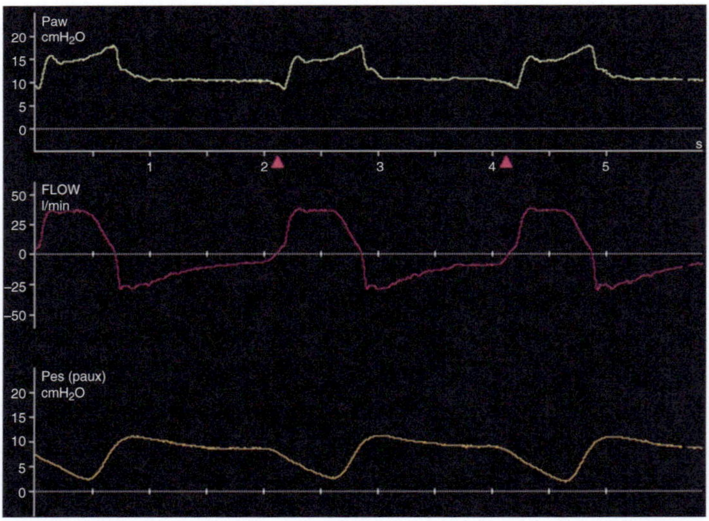

All statements are true except one. In a spontaneously breathing patient, P_{ES}:

1. Decreases at the beginning of inspiration
2. Increases during insufflation
3. Is lowest at the end of the inspiratory effort
4. Increases to baseline during the relaxation phase
5. Increases progressively during the relaxation phase

7.2.2 *Occlusion Test in Spontaneous Breathing Patient*

An occlusion test can be used to check the correct positioning of the esophageal balloon. An end-expiratory occlusion is performed. The patient develops a spontaneous inspiratory effort with closed airways. P_{AW} and P_{ES} decrease simultaneously during these efforts. The positioning is correct if the decrease in P_{AW} and P_{ES} is the same magnitude, i.e., *transpulmonary pressure remains stable during the occlusion test*. If this is not true, it usually means that P_{ES} is underestimating pleural pressure and transpulmonary (or trans-chest-wall) pressure calculations will be inaccurate (Video 7.16).

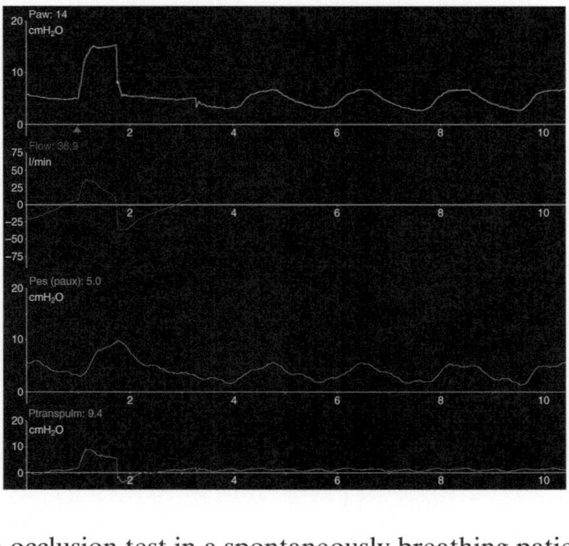

An occlusion test in a spontaneously breathing patient:

1. Is impossible to perform because the patient is not relaxed
2. Is performed by means of an end-expiratory occlusion
3. Is performed by observing the negative pressure swings in P_{AW} and P_{ES}
4. Is performed by monitoring transpulmonary pressure during an airway occlusion
5. All but 1

7.2.3 Transpulmonary Pressure

In spontaneously breathing patients, it is impossible to measure P_{TA} because P_{PLAT} can't be measured. However, it can be estimated based on transpulmonary pressure (P_{TP}), which is the difference between airway and esophageal pressure. Just as in passive patients, P_{TP} *should be limited to less than 20 cmH_2O* in spontaneously breathing patients to prevent lung injuries.

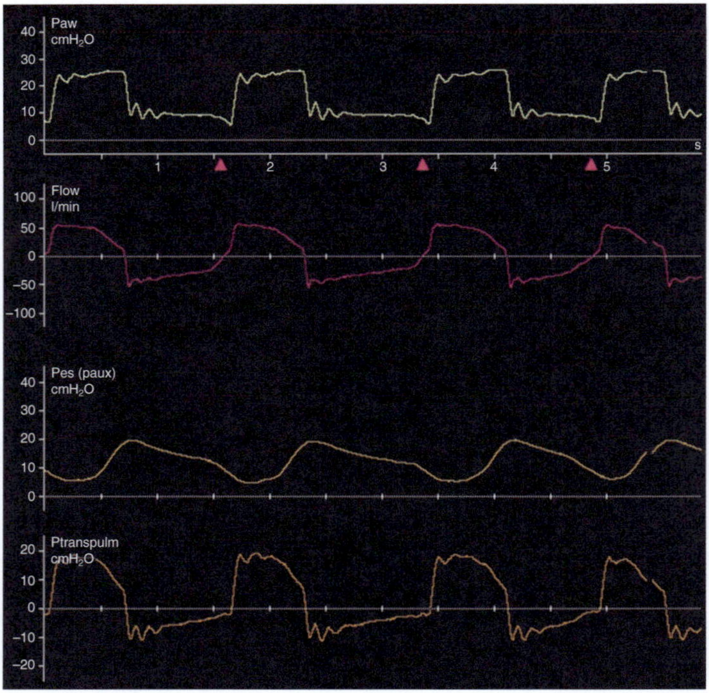

All statements regarding transpulmonary pressure are true *except*:

1. Transpulmonary pressure is used to assess transalveolar pressure in spontaneously breathing patients
2. Transpulmonary pressure is an overestimation of transalveolar pressure
3. Transpulmonary pressure is measured by means of an end-inspiratory and end-expiratory occlusion, respectively
4. Transpulmonary pressure is measured during ventilation with no occlusion
5. Transpulmonary pressure should be limited below 20 cmH_2O

7.2.4 Inspiratory Effort

The *shape of the decrease in P_{ES}* at the onset of the patient's inspiratory effort provides us with information about the *respiratory drive and the neuromuscular capacity*. A strong inspiratory effort is represented by a sharp, significant decrease in P_{ES}, while a weak effort is only small and gradual.

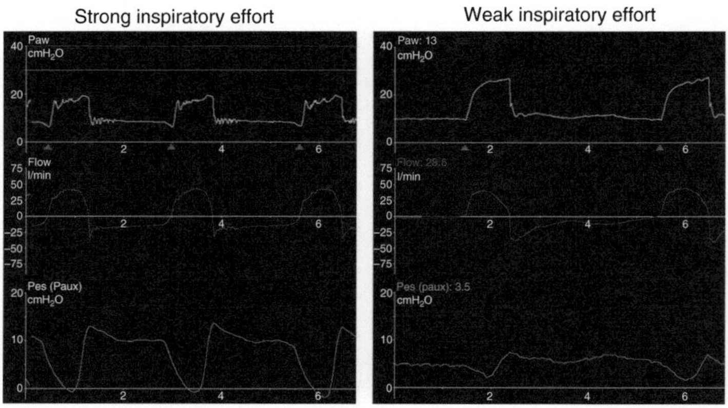

All statements regarding patient inspiratory effort are true *except*:

1. Can be assessed by the shape of the decrease in P_{ES}
2. Is different in each patient
3. Is the same for each breath in any one patient
4. Can be assessed by the size of the decrease in P_{ES}
5. Depends on the respiratory drive

7.2.5 *Shape of the Inspiratory Effort*

The decrease in P_{ES} demonstrates a change in slope. The initial decrease is steep, corresponding with the patient's effort before triggering the ventilator. The *change in slope occurs when the ventilator starts insufflation*. Subsequently, the inspiratory effort is weaker and inflation of the lung starts.

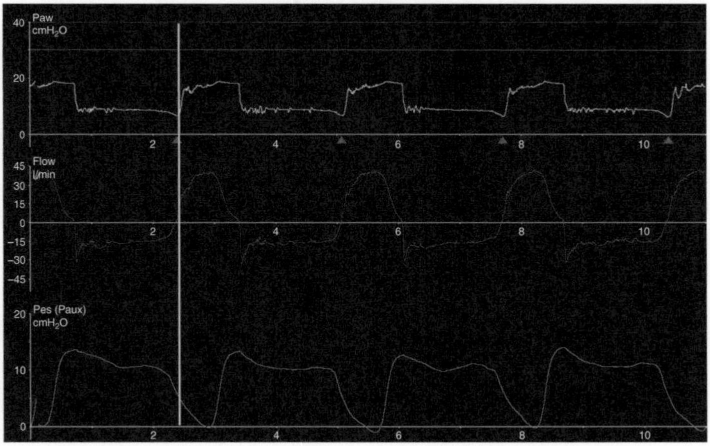

All statements are true except one. During inspiratory efforts, P_{ES}:

1. Decreases linearly
2. Decreases with a change in slope
3. Decreases rapidly before triggering the mechanical breath
4. Decreases more gradually after triggering the mechanical breath
5. Decreases more in the case of dynamic hyperinflation

7.2.6 Inspiratory Trigger Synchronization

Esophageal pressure shows the exact point where the patient's inspiratory effort starts. Delayed triggering occurs when the time between the start of the patient's effort and start of inspiratory pressure/flow is *longer than 200 ms*.

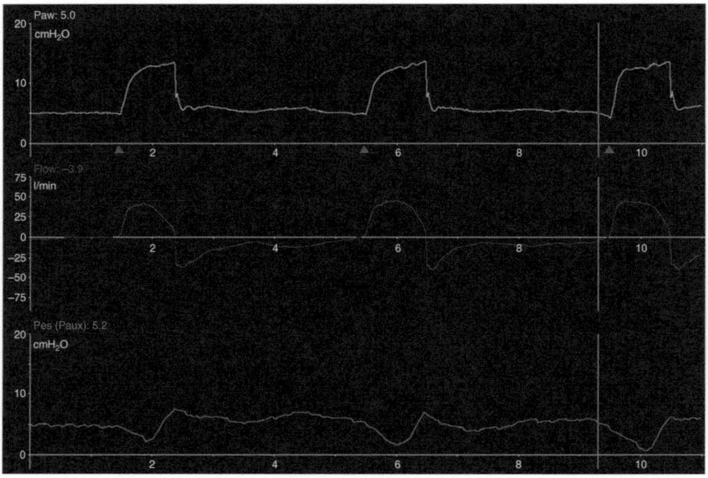

All statements regarding inspiratory trigger delay are true *except*:

1. Inspiratory trigger delay is measured from the beginning of the negative swing in P_{ES}
2. Inspiratory trigger delay depends on the respiratory drive
3. Inspiratory trigger delay depends on the rise time
4. Inspiratory trigger delay ends when airway pressure starts to increase
5. Inspiratory trigger delay depends on the inspiratory trigger setting

7.2.7 Ineffective Inspiratory Efforts

An ineffective inspiratory effort is shown as a *negative swing in P_{ES} that is not followed by flow crossing zero* (from expiration to inspiration). The inspiratory effort distorts airway flow and pressure as described in Sects. 4.1.6 and 5.7 (Video 7.17).

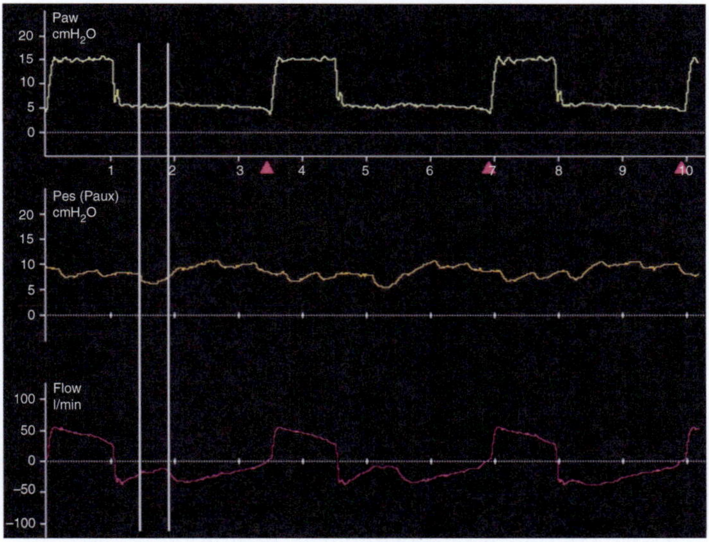

All statements are true except one. An ineffective inspiratory effort:

1. Is a negative swing in P_{ES} not followed by a mechanical breath
2. Occurs during expiration
3. Occurs near the end of a ventilator triggered breath
4. Can be interpreted as a cardiogenic oscillation
5. Is often associated with dynamic hyperinflation

7.2.8 Autotriggering

Autotriggering occurs when an assisted breath is triggered by the ventilator without the patient's inspiratory effort, i.e., in the *absence of a negative swing in* P_{ES}. Airway flow and pressure do not show the usual deflection before the start of inspiratory pressure/flow (Video 7.18).

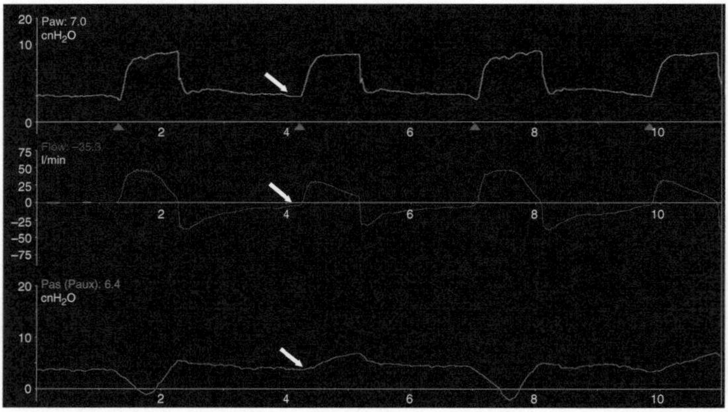

Autotriggering:

1. Occurs during at the beginning of expiration
2. Can be due to dynamic hyperinflation
3. Is equivalent to a ventilator triggered breath
4. Is a mechanical breath without the patient's inspiratory effort
5. Is associated with a weak respiratory drive

7.2.9 *Relaxation of Inspiratory Muscles*

Relaxation of the inspiratory muscles is indicated by the *return of P_{ES} to baseline*. It can be a sharp increase or a more gradual one. In many cases, there is an initial rapid change in P_{ES} followed by a more gradual change.

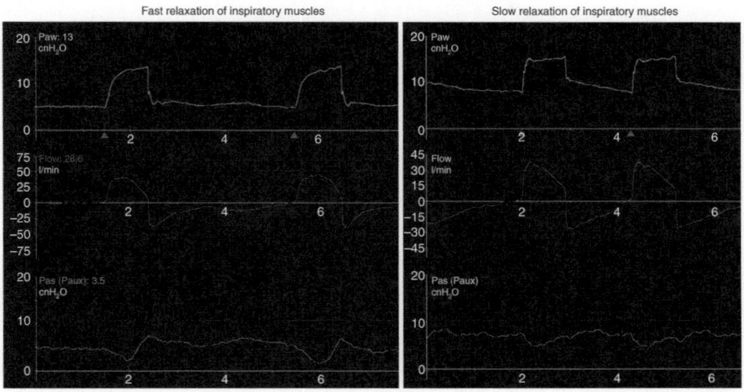

All statements are true except one. Relaxation of the inspiratory muscles:

1. Can be seen from the increase in P_{ES} to baseline
2. Has the same shape for all patients
3. Can change breath by breath in any one patient
4. Is shown by an initial rapid increase in P_{ES}, followed by a slow increase
5. Is distorted in the case of an active expiratory effort

7.2.10 Expiratory Trigger Synchronization

Mechanical insufflation should stop *near the middle point of inspiratory muscle relaxation*. If it stops earlier, this represents premature cycling. If it stops later, this represents delayed cycling. In both cases, airway flow and pressure show distortions as described in Sects. 4.1.18 and 4.1.19, respectively.

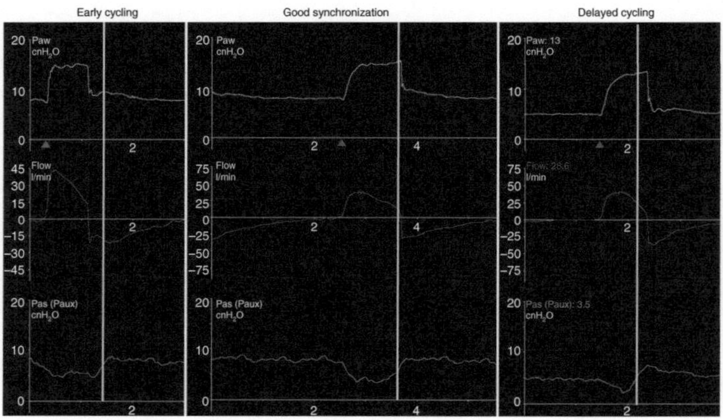

All statements regarding cycling are true *except*:

1. Cycling is the end of mechanical insufflation
2. Cycling has a significant impact on patient-ventilator synchrony
3. Cycling should occur at the end of the inspiratory effort
4. Cycling should occur in the middle of relaxation of the inspiratory muscles
5. Cycling is delayed when it occurs after the end of relaxation of the inspiratory muscles

7.2.11 *Passive Inflation and Active Expiratory Effort*

The shape of relaxation of the inspiratory effort is distorted in the case of passive inflation and active expiratory effort. Passive inflation occurs when the inspiratory effort is absent or is very short and weak relative to the inspiratory time. *P_{ES} increases as the lung is passively inflated.* P_{ES} may increase above the end-expiratory P_{ES} for a short period of time. An active expiratory effort is demonstrated by a sharp *increase in P_{ES} going above baseline.* This increase in P_{ES} above baseline is prolonged during expiration.

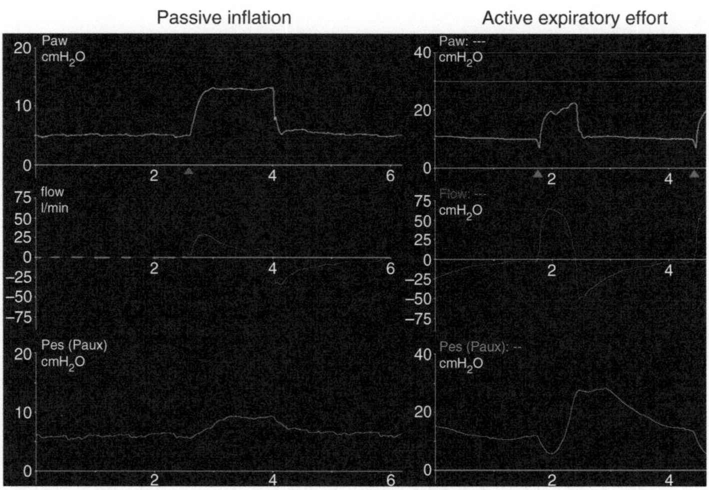

An increase in P_{ES} at the end of the inspiratory effort:

1. Is due to relaxation of the inspiratory muscles
2. Normally reaches the end-expiratory pressure
3. Can be distorted by an active expiratory effort
4. Can go above baseline
5. All above

Responses

7.1.1 3

7.1.2 2

7.1.3 5

7.1.4 1

7.1.5 1

7.1.6 1

7.1.7 4

7.1.8 5

7.1.9 1

7.1.10 5

7.1.11 2

7.1.12 3

7.1.13 2

7.1.14 5

7.2.1 2

7.2.2 5

7.2.3 3

7.2.4 3

7.2.5 1

7.2.6 3

7.2.7 3

3. This is a reverse triggering

4. The frequency of cardiogenic oscillation and ineffective inspiratory effort are different, but it is sometimes difficult to distinguish them when they are mixed

7.2.8 4

7.2.9 2

7.2.10 3

7.2.11 5

Suggested Readings

Akoumianaki E, Lyazidi A, et al. Mechanical ventilation-induced reverse-triggered breaths: a frequently unrecognized form of neuromechanical coupling. Chest. 2013;143:927–38.

Akoumianaki E, Maggiore SM, et al. The application of esophageal pressure measurement in patients with respiratory failure. Am J Respir Crit Care Med. 2014;189:520–31.

Baedorf Kassis E, Loring SH, et al. Mortality and pulmonary mechanics in relation to respiratory system and transpulmonary driving pressures in ARDS. Intensive Care Med. 2016;42:1206–13.

Baydur A, Behrakis PK, et al. A simple method for assessing the validity of the esophageal balloon technique. Am Rev Respir Dis. 1982;126:788–91.

Bellani G, Grasselli G, et al. Do spontaneous and mechanical breathing have similar effects on average transpulmonary and alveolar pressure? A clinical crossover study. Crit Care. 2016;20:142.

Benditt JO. Esophageal and gastric pressure measurements. Respir Care. 2005;50:6.

Chiumello D, Cressoni M, et al. The assessment of transpulmonary pressure in mechanically ventilated ARDS patients. Intensive Care Med. 2014;40:1670–8.

Chiumello D, Carlesso E, et al. Airway driving pressure and lung stress in ARDS patients. Crit Care. 2016a;20:276.

Chiumello D, Consonni D, et al. The occlusion tests and end-expiratory esophageal pressure: measurements and comparison in controlled and assisted ventilation. Ann Intensive Care. 2016b;6:13.

Kubiak BD, Gatto LA, et al. Plateau and transpulmonary pressure with elevated intra-abdominal pressure or atelectasis. J Surg Res. 2010;159:e17–24.

Loring SH, Topulos GP, et al. Transpulmonary Pressure: The Importance of Precise Definitions and Limiting Assumptions. Am J Respir Crit Care Med. 2016;194:1452–7.

Mauri T, Yoshida T, et al. Esophageal and transpulmonary pressure in the clinical setting: meaning, usefulness and perspectives. Intensive Care Med. 2016;42:1360–73.

Mojoli F, Chiumello D, et al. Esophageal pressure measurements under different conditions of intrathoracic pressure. An in vitro study of second generation balloon catheters. Minerva Anestesiol. 2015;81:855–64.

Mojoli F, Iotti GA, et al. In vivo calibration of esophageal pressure in the mechanically ventilated patient makes measurements reliable. Crit Care. 2016;20:98.

Sahetya SK, Brower RG. The promises and problems of transpulmonary pressure measurements in acute respiratory distress syndrome. Curr Opin Crit Care. 2016;22:7–13.

Talmor D, Sarge T, et al. Esophageal and transpulmonary pressures in acute respiratory failure. Crit Care Med. 2006;34:1389–94.

Talmor D, Sarge T, et al. Mechanical ventilation guided by esophageal pressure in acute lung injury. N Engl J Med. 2008;359:2095–104.

Terragni P, Mascia L, et al. Accuracy of esophageal pressure to assess transpulmonary pressure during mechanical ventilation. Intensive Care Med. 2017;43:142–3.

Yonis H, Gobert F, et al. Reverse triggering in a patient with ARDS. Intensive Care Med. 2015;41:1711–2.

MIX
Papier aus verantwortungsvollen Quellen
Paper from responsible sources
FSC® C105338

If you have any concerns about our products,
you can contact us on
ProductSafety@springernature.com

In case Publisher is established outside the EU,
the EU authorized representative is:
Springer Nature Customer Service Center GmbH
Europaplatz 3, 69115 Heidelberg, Germany

Printed by Libri Plureos GmbH
in Hamburg, Germany